Contents

Thanks and acknowledgements

The authors and publishers would like to thank the following institutions and teachers for their help in piloting and commenting on the material and for the invaluable feedback which they provided:

Alison Ridley, The Hong Kong Polytechnic University, Hong Kong; Anne Dorey, EF International, Sydney, Australia; Robert Turner, UNESCO Hanoi, Vietnam; Emma Levy, English Language Teaching Centre, New Delhi, India; Havovi Kolsawalla, British Council Division, Mumbai, India.

The sample answer sheets on page 4 and pages 103–108 are reproduced by kind permission of the University of Cambridge Local Examinations Syndicate.

The cassette which accompanies this book was recorded by Martin Williamson at Studio AVP in London.

6-50

Practice Tests for the Cambridge Business English Certificate Level 2

Jake Allsop
Patricia Aspinall

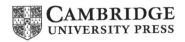

CAMBRIDGE
UNIVERSITY PRESS

PUBLISHED BY THE PRESS SYNDICATE OF THE UNIVERSITY OF CAMBRIDGE
The Pitt Building, Trumpington Street, Cambridge, United Kingdom

CAMBRIDGE UNIVERSITY PRESS
The Edinburgh Building, Cambridge CB2 2RU, United Kingdom   www.cup.cam.ac.uk
40 West 20th Street, New York, NY 10011–4211, USA   www.cup.org
10 Stamford Road, Oakleigh, Melbourne 3166, Australia
Ruiz de Alarcón 13, 28014 Madrid, Spain

First published 1999

Printed in the United Kingdom at the University Press, Cambridge

ISBN 0 521 648483 Book
ISBN 0 521 64447X Cassette

Introduction

TO THE STUDENT

This book is for people who are going to take the Business English Certificate Level 2 (BEC 2).

About the BEC examinations

The University of Cambridge Local Examinations Syndicate (UCLES) Business English Certificate (BEC) examinations offer an English language qualification for learners who want to use English for international business. All the material in the examinations is based on real-world business situations. There are three levels: BEC 1, BEC 2 and BEC 3.

About BEC 2

BEC 2 is for candidates with English at the intermediate level who are one of the following: students preparing for a career in business; those already in business at the lower to middle management levels; middle and senior clerical staff.

Note: For a more detailed explanation of the BEC examinations, teachers should refer to the Teacher's Handbook and other BEC documentation, available from UCLES.

About this book

This book is for candidates preparing for the BEC 2 examination. The aims of the book are:
- to give you practice in doing the BEC 2 examination
- to make you familiar with the texts, topics, tasks and test formats that you will meet in the examination
- to show you the level and kind of language tested in the BEC 2 examination.

Contents of the book

It contains the following:
- four complete practice BEC 2 examinations
- sample photocopiable OMR Answer Sheets
- transcripts of all the Listening material
- answer keys for the Reading and Listening tests
- sample answers for the Writing tests.

The accompanying 90-minute audio cassette contains four Listening tests and a complete example of the Speaking test.

The examination format

The BEC 2 examination consists of three tests – Reading and Writing, Listening and Speaking – and is completed in two stages as shown on the following page.

The Reading and Writing test

The **Reading** section of the test uses different kinds of texts with a business theme, including graphics, e.g. descriptions of products, job advertisements, newspaper articles and reports.

The **Writing** section of the test consists of two tasks. In the first task you are asked to write a note, message or memo and include three specific pieces of information given in the instructions. In the second task you are asked to produce an extended piece of writing such as a business letter or report.

Marking Parts 1 and 2 of the Writing test

For **Part 1**, you can get full marks (i.e. 10 marks) if you have communicated all three parts of the message in an appropriate style, and if your English is easy to understand and has no serious mistakes in it.

For **Part 2**, you can get full marks (i.e. 15

Stage One	Reading and Writing	50 minutes	6 parts, 45 marks	
			Part 1 - four information texts, matching task	7 marks
			Part 2 - single text, matching task	5 marks
			Part 3 - single text, multiple matching	8 marks
			Part 4 - single informational text, multiple choice	15 marks
			Part 5a - short text, error correction	5 marks
			Part 5b - short text, error correction	5 marks
		40 minutes	2 parts, 25 marks	
			Part 1 - note or memo	10 marks
			Part 2 - letter or report	15 marks
	Listening	40 minutes	3 parts, 30 marks	
			Part 1 - three telephone messages of conversations	12 marks
			Part 2 - 10 short monologues	10 marks
			Part 3 - an extended conversation/monologue	8 marks
Stage Two	Speaking	12 minutes (18 minutes for for 3 candidates)	Part 1 - interview with the examiner Part 2 - communication task with another candidate	

marks) if you covered all the points of information required, wrote a text of the correct length and if your answer was in an appropriate style, easy to understand, well-planned, and with a good use of vocabulary and tenses.

The Listening test

The **Listening** test uses different kinds of spoken texts with a business theme, e.g. messages, monologues, interviews, conversations and discussions. You hear each text twice. In the examination, at the end of the test, you are given 10 minutes to transfer your answers on to the OMR sheet.

For the Listening test, you have to:
- find the information from three short spoken texts and fill in three gapped texts
- match 10 (2 × 5) short texts to a set of items
- answer eight multiple choice questions on a longer spoken text.

Note: When working with the audio cassette which accompanies this book, you will need to rewind in order to hear each text twice.

Marking the Listening test

Each correct answer is given 1 mark. There are no half marks.

Speaking

The **Speaking** section of the test is an interview with two candidates (sometimes three candidates). There are two examiners: one examiner (the interlocutor) will talk to the candidates, and the other examiner just listens.

The test is in two parts. In Part 1 you have to talk about yourself. This part of the test lasts 3–4 minutes.

In Part 2 you have to find out information you need to complete a task. You and the other candidate are given 'activity sheets' which tell you what you have to talk to each other about. You have 30 seconds to read through your sheet and 2 minutes to ask and answer questions. In the Sample Speaking Test on the cassette, you can hear two candidates taking part in Speaking Test 1.

Marking the Speaking test

You are given a mark between 0 and 3 according to how well you used grammar and vocabulary; how well you organised what you said; how clear your pronunciation was; how well you worked with your partner.

Both examiners will mark you, and this will result in a final grade of 1, 2 or 3 (where 1 is the highest).

What is the pass mark for the examination?

For Stage 1 (Reading/Writing and Listening), you are awarded a grade: A, B, C, D or E. Only candidates with grades A–D will receive a BEC Certificate. In percentage terms, the pass marks at each grade are roughly as follows:
A 80+% B 70–79% C 60–69% D 50–59% E less than 50%.

For Stage 2 (Speaking), you are awarded a separate grade: 1, 2 or 3. Grades 1 and 2 are added to the BEC certificate. For grade 3, the words 'No Grade' for Speaking are added to your certificate.

How to use the OMR Answer Sheets

In the BEC 2 examination, you will write your answers on OMR Answer Sheets (see pp. 103–108). Use a 2B pencil, have an eraser to erase any mistakes.

The OMR is divided into three sections:
- the **first (top) section** is for your examination number
- the **second section** is for entering your answers to the Reading section
- the **third section** is for entering your answers to the Writing section.

Enter your response by shading out the appropriate square. If you make a mistake, erase the incorrect response and then enter the correct response.

Important note: If you enter more than one answer to a question, you will get no marks for that question, even if one of the answers is correct.

You write complete words, numbers or sentences in this section. Do not shade out the squares.

Enter your responses by writing the word(s), numbers or sentences on the lines provided.

TO THE TEACHER

The preceding notes to the student give an outline of the different parts of the BEC 2 exam, including information on the mark allocation and on using the OMR (Optical Mark Reader) sheet. UCLES makes past question papers available for a fee. Please contact UCLES centres for details.

The Speaking test

The speaking tests in this book give your students the chance to familiarise themselves with the structure and procedure of the test, and to learn what to expect and how to perform under interview conditions. If you test the students on your own, make them aware that there are always two examiners present in the real examination. They should also be made aware they might do the test in a group of three (although the communication activity will only be with one other student).

Notes on conducting the Speaking test

The test is in two parts. In Part 1 you ask each student about themselves. Ask each student slightly different questions. Sometimes it is possible to ask a student two or three consecutive questions, but try to make sure that each student has the same number of questions. This part of the test lasts 3–4 minutes. The aim is to test the student on their ability to give personal information about themselves, their homes, interests and jobs and to show that they can agree or disagree and express preferences.

In Part 2 there are two communication activities for the students. Give the students time to read through their activity sheets, so they understand what they have to do, and then each student in turn asks the other student three questions using the prompts on their sheets. Each student has 2 minutes to complete the questioning task.

The activity sheets lead into a short discussion on the topic. The discussion topic is given on the activity sheets. Give the students about 30 seconds to prepare for the discussion. They should not make any notes. The discussion lasts about 3 minutes.

This book contains four practice speaking tests, showing the kind of questions that you can ask the students in the test. The Speaking test from

Test 1 is also recorded on the cassette as an example.

Marking the Speaking test

BEC 2 examiners give candidates a mark for each of the following criteria and for overall performance:

- pronunciation:
  control of both individual sounds and prosodic features such as stress, rhythm and intonation
- grammar and vocabulary:
  accuracy and appropriacy of candidate's structures and vocabulary
- discourse management:
  ability to use English beyond sentence level: coherence and organisation, fluency over several utterances, appropriate complexity of structures
- interactive communication:
  ability to interact, taking turns, imitating and responding, positively contributing, amount of assistance required.

The marks for these criteria are translated into total scores, which are then graded. Use these grade descriptors:

Pronunciation
5 easy to understand
3 occasionally difficult to understand
1 sometimes difficult to understand

Grammar and vocabulary
5 meaning is conveyed with few errors
3 meaning is conveyed with some minor errors
1 meaning is generally conveyed, despite errors

Discourse management
5 no strain on the listener
3 occasional strain on the listener
1 some strain on listener

Interactive communication
5 independent communicator
3 fairly independent communicator
1 sometimes dependent

Marking Parts 1 and 2 of the Writing test

Part 1, question 46, requires candidates to write a memo of about 40 words. Typically, candidates get full marks if they provide all the required information, and in language which is free of serious errors. Candidates should be careful not to exceed the recommended number of words.

Part 2, question 47, requires candidates to produce a continuous piece of writing, usually about 120 words, often in the form of a report or letter. Typically, candidates are awarded marks for their performance in two areas: completion of the task, i.e. content, and quality of language. It is important not to exceed the recommended number of words.

Test 1

READING AND WRITING   1 hour 30 minutes

READING

Questions 1–45

PART ONE

Questions 1–7

- Look at the sentences below and the job advertisements on page 6.
- Which job does each sentence **1–7** refer to?
- For each sentence, mark **one** letter **A**, **B**, **C** or **D** on your Answer Sheet.
- You will need to use some of the letters more than once.

Example:	**Answer**
You will need to know a foreign language for this job.	
	A **B** **C** **D**

1 You could get this job without having a degree or diploma.

2 You must have a science degree for this job. ⁄|

3 If you are interested in this job, you should send for an application form.

4 They want to know how much you are earning in your present job.

5 Your letter of application should not be typewritten.

6 The company wants you to tell them how much you want to earn with them.

7 This job is a management position.

A

> **Medical Representative** to sell pharmaceutical products to doctors and pharmacists. You need to have a science degree, experience in sales/marketing, and an ability to get on with people. The job offers an excellent salary, employee benefits and opportunities for career advancement. Apply in writing, with CV and expected salary.

B

> **Senior Training Officer (Technical)** to take charge of Bukit Vehicle Maintenance Training Centre. The job involves running the Centre, providing in-house staff training and updating present programmes. An engineering degree and previous experience of the automotive industry are essential. Send career details with photograph and three professional references.

C

> **Lecturers** for the Singapore Excellence Institute to teach Tourism, Business Management or Media Studies. The posts are part-time, but could become permanent after one year. Candidates need a degree or diploma in a relevant subject and five years' teaching experience. Send CV with covering handwritten letter and details of current salary.

D

> **Executive Officer (Payment)** to supervise payment operations. You must be fluent in English and Mandarin, familiar with computer operations, and have a qualification in accounting or three years' relevant experience. We offer a competitive salary, generous holiday allowance, bonus scheme and free medical insurance. For further details and an application form, phone or write to Personnel Officer, Jurong Ltd.

PART TWO

Questions 8–12

- Read the text below about videoconferencing.
- Choose the best sentence from page 8 to fill in each of the gaps.
- For each gap **8–12**, mark one letter **A–I** on your Answer Sheet.
- Do not use any letter more than once.

In this technological age, you no longer need to spend long hours in the car or waiting around at airports just to attend routine meetings. **(example)** ....

Videoconferencing uses a system that incorporates a remote control mini-camera and microphone, a screen and loudspeakers for easy two-way communication. **(8)** ....

There are many ways in which you can use this new technology. **(9)** ....

The vision of the travel-free corporation is, of course, as unrealistic as the paper-free office. **(10)** ....

Indeed, the forecast is that the videoconferencing market is now growing at a rate of 166% p.a. **(11)** ....

Then, videoconferencing systems were very specialised and cost in the region of £250,000. **(12)** ....

As prices tumble further over the next couple of years, visual communications will become a routine facility like fax, word processing or e-mail.

example:	A B C D E F G H I
	☐ ☐ ☐ ☐ ☐ ☐ ■ ☐ ☐

A In addition, it enables senior managers to become more involved in subsidiaries and to control worldwide operations from head office.

B Ten years ago, such growth would have seemed impossible.

C Clearly, a number of companies are finding that the investment is worth it.

D By providing a live link between two or more locations, videoconferencing enables from 2 to 200 people to see, hear and talk to each other and to present, look at and discuss documents together.

E Today, by contrast, the equivalent systems cost about one-tenth of that, with mobile systems like the BT VC7000 now on offer at under £6,000.

F Until now, videoconferencing was only possible via expensive fixed digital links (private leased lines) between two locations.

G You could, instead, hold a videoconference.

H However, just as fax swept through the office in the 1980s, so videoconferencing will be the new application for office-to-office communications by the year 2000.

I They include weekly sales meetings, customer presentations, sales and service training, staff announcements and financial reviews.

PART THREE

Questions 13–20

- Read this text about the changing role of Asian women.
- Answer questions **13–20** on page 10.

Rising power of women in Asia

Although most still live by centuries-old traditions, millions of professional Asian women will enter the twenty-first century as a force the entire world must reckon with. Educated and business-minded, they are demanding a full partnership with men, and playing a leading role in the economic explosion of the Pacific Rim. A new generation of women is taking top positions in the family business or launching new businesses financed by the family.

1. It is true, of course, that Asia's women leaders are a privileged class, and there is a great difference between urban and rural women. Still, the patterns that will change the lives of hundreds of millions of Asian women are already in place. These professional women are well educated. In Taiwan, for example, women aged 20–24 match the college graduation rates of their male counterparts.

2. And yet Asia's quiet women-led revolution is not simply the story of women managers. It is also the story of ordinary women – peasant farmers and labourers. Asia's economic miracle would not have been possible without their participation. For example, Korea's industrial base was built by a legion of women working at repetitive dead-end and poorly-paid jobs in the electronics, textile and toy factories. Similarly, in Malaysia, thousands of rural women migrated to the cities to work in the electronic factories, thus helping to transform a largely agriculture-based economy to one that is rapidly industrialising.

3. Amongst the causes of this revolution, the principal one is opportunity. Asia's exploding economy and the small populations of some Asian countries (Singapore has only 3 million people) mean labour shortages and full employment. Business must make use of all human resources. In addition, many international companies with branches in Asia are accustomed to hiring women.

4. Equally important is the fact that modern Asian women are not like their mothers. Not only are they better educated than their mothers, but they are also marrying later, if at all, and having fewer children. Moreover, the Asian woman today is much better informed. Instant access to global events via international broadcast systems gives her a window on the world that earlier generations knew nothing about. And in the workplace, the new technology is 'gender-blind', that is, there is nothing in it which makes it more suitable for men than for women.

Questions 13–16

- For questions **13–16**, choose from the list **A–G** the best title for each numbered paragraph in the text.
- For each numbered paragraph **1–4**, mark **one** letter **A–G** on your Answer Sheet.
- Do not use any letter more than once.

13 Paragraph 1 ....

14 Paragraph 2 ....

15 Paragraph 3 ....

16 Paragraph 4 ....

A The new Asian woman
B Traditional values
C The population explosion
D The importance of education
E The exploding demand for labour
F Modern women in a changing world
G The role of uneducated women

Questions 17–20

- Using the information in the text, complete each sentence **17–20** with a phrase **A–G** from the list below.
- For each sentence **17–20**, mark **one** letter **A–G** on your Answer Sheet.
- Do not use any letter more than once.

17 The small size of some Asian countries means that ....

18 Many women are able to start up new businesses because ....

19 A consequence of educated women having smaller families is that ....

20 Asian women are well informed nowadays because ....

A there are plenty of jobs for everyone
B they are free to pursue their careers
C the work is more suitable for women
D their families provide the money
E the government wants more women to become managers
F they have access to world news through the media
G they have more political power nowadays

PART FOUR

Questions 21–35

- Read this article about a new fund in India.
- Choose the correct word from **A, B, C** or **D** on page 12 to fill in each gap.
- For each question **21–35**, mark **one** letter **A, B, C** or **D** on your Answer Sheet.

Financial help for Indian companies

A $160 million project to make the 'Made in India' label better known abroad has just been announced in New Delhi. The 'Brand Equity Fund', as it is called, is a project backed by India's federal government to (**example**) .... Indian companies a foothold in the world market. It is the first ever government (**21**) .... of its type.

A government spokesman announced that the fund would be (**22**) .... in the next few days, and would help Indian companies to (**23**) .... specific brands.
But business people are (**24**) .... about the scheme's likely benefits. Critics say that not enough money has been put into the fund to make it really (**25**) .... They say that the (**26**) .... is too little to help the tens of thousands of small Indian companies whose limited (**27**) .... prevent them from making a serious impact on international markets.

India's economy was once (**28**) .... closed to foreign investment, but it opened up to foreign companies five or so years ago under sweeping reforms (**29**) .... by the former Prime Minister, Mr P V Narasimha Rao. The moves have so far (**30**) .... more than $20 billion worth of foreign investment.

But, although certain Indian (**31**) .... , such as Darjeeling tea, upmarket silk, leather, cotton, gem stones and jewellery do quite well, no single Indian brand has yet (**32**) .... the top rank. The fund is a serious (**33**) .... to change this. The government (**34**) .... , however, that brands selected for promotion abroad should be of international quality and (**35**) .... of making a real impact in the global market.

Test 1

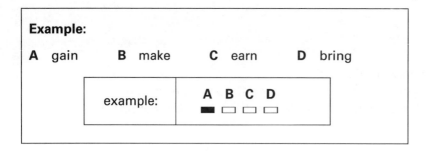
21 A function   B event   C advertisement   D campaign

22 A launched   B fired   C pronounced   D started

23 A invent   B promote   C support   D develop

24 A doubtful   B worried   C suspicious   D unhappy

25 A definite   B certain   C effective   D valuable

26 A addition   B quantity   C amount   D size

27 A properties   B stocks   C companies   D resources

28 A completely   B utterly   C absolutely   D particularly

29 A provided   B required   C introduced   D discovered

30 A claimed   B encouraged   C persuaded   D attracted

31 A products   B types   C industries   D names

32 A brought   B reached   C obtained   D performed

33 A trial   B attempt   C concern   D business

34 A declares   B reserves   C presumes   D insists

35 A confident   B worthy   C capable   D aware

PART FIVE

Section A

Questions 36–40

- Read this letter about a wrong order.
- In most of the lines **36–40** there is **one extra word** which does not fit. One or two lines, however, are correct.
- If a line is correct, put a tick (✔) in the space on your Answer Sheet.
- If there is an extra word in the line, write that word in the space on your Answer Sheet.

Examples:

We should like to apologise for the delay, and can assure you that   .... ✔ ....

such as a thing will not happen again.   .... *as* ....

Dear Mrs Starling

Thank you for your letter of 8 March. We are sorry that the valve

36   we sent you for was the wrong size. It seems that our suppliers no

37   longer stock 50 mm valves. Our shipping clerk did not notice so that

38   the valve was the wrong specification. We have found an alternative

39   supplier, who they have 50 mm valves in stock. These valves are

40   very more expensive than those stocked by our previous supplier, but

we will supply a replacement valve at the old price.

Yours sincerely

PART FIVE

Section B

Questions 41–45

- A colleague of yours has written a memo and has asked you to check it.
- In each line there is **one wrong word**.
- For each line **41–45**, write the **correct word** in the space on your Answer Sheet.

Examples:

When you application for a job, always send a covering letter with your CV. .... *apply* ....

Your letter should be neat written. .... *neatly* ....

Computer Workstation

The base unit and monitor rest neatly on the desktop. Below this,

41 there is a keyboard shelf. The shelf pulls out when your using

42 the keyboard. When the keyboard is not in use, you can pushing

43 the shelf back under the desktop. This shelf also have a built-in

44 wrist rest to provide comfortable and support while you are typing.

45 The desk has an adjustable foot rest and the chair what is

supplied with the workstation provides support for the lower back.

WRITING

Questions 46 and 47

PART ONE

Question 46

- You work in a company which deals with industrial waste. You have read about a new kind of pump which could save your company thousands of dollars in servicing and maintenance costs.
- Write a memo of **30–40 words** to your Head of Department saying:
  - where you read about the new pump
  - why you think it could be a good investment
  - how you might get more information about it.
- **Write on your Answer Sheet.**

PART TWO

Question 47

● You are the secretary at the Birmingham branch of CADE Hazards. Your boss has asked you to organise a one-day conference. You sent this memo to the Conference Organiser, and received her memo in reply.

1   Your memo to the Conference Organiser.

To: Conference Organiser, CADE Group Head Office, London

From: Secretary, CADE Hazards, Birmingham

Date: 23.04.99

Re: Arrangements for CADE Hazards one-day Conference

Please let me know if you can make arrangements based on the following:

Venue - Preferably Natt Conference Centre, Itching, Herts.

Date - 5 June 1999

Times - Registration 08.30–09.00. First session 09.15. Last session scheduled to end at 16.30

Number attending - Estimated 40

Room requirements - Main conference hall with usual audiovisual facilities + 4 side rooms for small group meetings.

Travel - Contact Sid's Cabs for transfers from Itching station to Conference Centre

Food, etc. - Arrange coffee and tea mid-morning and mid-afternoon, buffet lunch (check on arrangements for vegetarians)

Other - Check if any participants require overnight accommodation and arrange with Natt (Company will pay room and breakfast only)

---

2   This is the Conference Organiser's reply.

i	Natt available only 4 June in that week. Change date of conference or find a different venue?
ii	Natt can do conference rooms, refreshments, lunch (incl. vegetarian). Need to know exact numbers by 30 May.
iii	Five delegates need accommodation. No residential accommodation at Natt, but local hotel has vacancies (advance payment required).
iv	Travel: all participants coming by car, except 5. Two taxis arranged with Sid's Cabs (who pays?).

3   You also received this note from your boss.

As this month is the tenth anniversary of the founding of the CADE group of companies, we should arrange some kind of a dinner in the evening after the conference.

- Write a report of **100–120 words** to the Head Office Conference Organiser telling her what you have finally decided about the arrangements for the conference, including the evening dinner. Use the information in the documents above.
- **Write on your Answer Sheet.**

LISTENING   Approximately 40 minutes (including 10 minutes transfer time)

PART ONE

Questions 1–12

- You will hear three recorded telephone messages.
- Write **one** or **two** words or a number in the numbered spaces on the forms below.
- After each message, rewind the tape and listen again.

Message One
(Questions 1–4)

- Look at the form below.
- You will hear a man leaving a message for his bank.

Caller: Lewis Bradfield
Firm: Collings (**1**) .... Company
Date: Tuesday, 14 February
Time of call: (**2**) ....

Has received his (**3**) .... with several

(**4**) .... he is unsure about.

Please ring him as soon as possible.

Message Two
(Questions 5–8)

- Look at the form below.
- You will hear a hotel manager leaving a message for Mr Lacey.

Caller: The Mandarin Court Hotel, Shanghai
Date and time: 8.6.98 @ 8 a.m.

Hotel confirms booking for Mr Lacey. Expect him to arrive on 12 June. Reservation is until (**5**) ....

He has been put in a (**6**) .... room on the 14th floor as requested.

Room rate offered $ (**7**) ....

Fax/phone no. is 86 21 (**8**) ....

**Message Three
(Questions 9–12)**

- Look at the form below.
- You will hear a man from a computer rental company leaving a message.

Caller:	Computer Rental Services
Date and time of message:	10.30 a.m., 27 November

Confirms that a (**9**) .... computer is available for rent.

Cost: $ (**10**) .... per month plus insurance. (Taking out of country?)

Please advise on (**11**) .... date.

Call Jim Darma on (**12**) .... today, if possible.

PART TWO

Questions 13–22

**Section One
(Questions 13–17)**

- You will hear five people talking about different items.
- For each piece, decide which item **A–H** the speaker is talking about.
- Write **one** letter **A–H** next to the number of the piece.
- Do not use any letter more than once.
- At the end of question 17, rewind the tape and listen again.

13 ....

14 ....

15 ....

16 ....

17 ....

A photocopier
B hotel booking
C expenses claim
D meeting
E fax machine
F advertisements
G report
H business plan

Section Two
(Questions 18–22)

- You will hear another five short pieces.
- For each piece, decide who the speaker is.
- Write **one** letter **A–H** next to the number of the piece.
- Do not use any letter more than once.
- At the end of question 22, rewind the tape and listen again.

18 ....

19 ....

20 ....

21 ....

22 ....

A secretary
B telephone engineer
C security guard
D hotel receptionist
E bank manager
F builder
G conference delegate
H waiter

PART THREE

Questions 23–30

- You will hear a woman giving advice on how to give a good presentation.
- Choose the best phrase to answer or complete questions **23–30**.
- Mark **one** letter **A, B** or **C** for the sentence you choose.
- At the end of the talk, rewind the tape and listen again.

23 How should you stand when giving a presentation?

    A   keep your knees straight
    B   keep your head still
    C   keep your feet apart

24 What happens if you stick your neck forwards?

    A   your throat will get sore
    B   your voice will sound strange
    C   your head will feel light

25 What should you do if you are nervous?

    A   examine your feelings
    B   make detailed notes
    C   go for a massage

26 What can you do to make your presentation sound more interesting?

    A speak loudly and clearly
    B sound enthusiastic
    C ask the audience questions

27 Which body type might an audience find irritating?

    A passive
    B aggressive
    C assertive

28 What is characteristic of an aggressive body type?

    A playing with hair
    B swinging leg
    C clear voice

29 What should you avoid doing before a presentation?

    A drinking coffee
    B eating too much
    C smoking

30 If you have a cold, remember to

    A clear your throat before speaking.
    B use your tongue and lips more.
    C drink small amounts of alcohol.

**You now have 10 minutes to transfer your answers
to your Answer Sheet.**

SPEAKING   Approximately 12 minutes

Ordering products
*For **two** candidates*

Candidate A

YOUR QUESTIONS

In this activity you will find out information about two types of overhead projector
(OHP). You will then discuss with your partner which one you are going to buy.
First find out more about the Novo Overhead Projector. Ask candidate B your
questions.

1	Price:	....
2	Weight:	....
3	Extra features:	....

Discussion:

Discuss with your partner what makes the projector the most suitable for you.
Consider **price** and **weight** and any other features you think are important.

INFORMATION

Your partner will ask you questions about the Casco Executive Projector. Use the
information below to answer the questions.

Casco Executive Overhead Projector

- Compact but strong with fold down arm for easy storage
- Weight: 10.8 kg
- Economy lamp circuit
- Twin fan cooling system
- Pack includes LCD projection panel, Universal Power Supply, Remote Control
  Unit and User Manual
- Price: £600.00   Product Code: 154712[C]

Ordering products
*For **two** candidates*

Candidate B

YOUR QUESTIONS

In this activity you will find out information about two types of overhead projector (OHP). You will then discuss with your partner which one you are going to buy. First find out more about the Casco Executive Overhead Projector. Ask candidate A your questions.

1 Size: ....

2 Instructions for use: ....

3 Extra features: ....

Discussion:

Discuss with your partner what makes the projector the most suitable for you. Consider **price** and **weight** and any other features you think are important.

INFORMATION

Your partner will ask you questions about the Novo Overhead Projector. Use the information below to answer the questions.

The Novo Overhead Projector

- Portable and lightweight (5.6 kg)
- Folds flat for travelling
- Storage carrying case
- Overall size: 330 x 430 x 210
- Twin lamps
- Price: £497.50   Product Code: 366242 [E]

Test 2

READING AND WRITING   1 hour 30 minutes

Questions 1–45

PART ONE

Questions 1–7

- Read these sentences and the four sets of office regulations on the opposite page.
- Which set of regulations does each sentence **1–7** refer to?
- For each sentence, mark **one** letter **A, B, C** or **D** on your Answer Sheet.
- You will need to use some of these letters more than once.

<table>
<tr><td>Example:</td><td>Answer</td></tr>
<tr><td>Load the paper tray whenever you use the machine.</td><td>■   □   □   □
A   B   C   D</td></tr>
</table>

1 Tell the person in charge if anyone is not at work on that day.

2 The time allowed for this is one hour.

3 Tell your boss before you go to this place.

4 This is not for your own private use.

5 This tells you the actions you must take in the interests of safety.

6 Tell the appropriate person if there is a mechanical problem.

7 These are the times when you must be at your place of work.

A

> **Rules for use of photocopier**
> Please enter in the log the following information every time you use the photocopier:
>   date, name and department, number of passes, number of sheets of paper used.
> Use of the machine for copying personal documents is strictly forbidden.
> In the event of a breakdown, switch off the machine and inform the Office Manager
>   immediately.
> Make sure that the paper tray is loaded before and after you use the machine.

B

> **Fire Drill**
> There will be a fire drill at 10.30 on the second Tuesday of every month.
> When you hear the fire alarm, immediately stop what you are doing.
> Close all the windows and close the door when you leave your office.
> Walk to the assembly point outside the building (see map).
> Report to the Fire Drill Officer and inform him/her if any of your colleagues are absent.
> Do not re-enter the building until told to do so.

C

> **Use of Sick Room**
> The Sick Room is only to be used in genuine cases of illness or injury.
> If you are ill or have an accident, inform your immediate superior before going to the
>   Sick Room.
> The Nurse will give emergency treatment only.
> Normally, a visit to the sick room should not last more than thirty minutes.
> In case of serious illness or injury, employees will be sent or taken to hospital.

D

> **Flexitime**
> Employees may start work at any time between 07.00 and 09.30, and finish not earlier
>   than 16.30 and not later than 18.00.
> The one-hour lunch break must be taken between 12.00 and 14.00.
> Thus, 'block times' (i.e. when all employees are in) are 09.30 – 12.00 and 14.00 – 16.30.
> Employees must agree their flexitime arrangements with their immediate superior.

PART TWO

Questions 8–12

- Read this text about 'intranets'.
- Choose the best sentence from the opposite page to fill in each of the gaps.
- For each gap **8–12**, mark one letter **A–I** on your Answer Sheet.
- Do not use any letter more than once.

Everybody has heard about the **Internet**, but do you know what an '**intranet**' is? (**example**) ....

In fact, intranets make use of the same software programs as the Internet to connect computers and people. (**8**) ....

If your intranet is working properly, it can link together huge amounts of information which is stored in different places in the company. (**9**) ....

A company intranet can, of course, be used for unimportant information like office memos and canteen menus. (**10**) ....

The intranet is a great idea, but the system only works if everyone on the intranet is willing to share their information with other people. (**11**) ....

Another problem which often occurs is that top managers like to use the intranet to 'communicate down' rather than to 'communicate across'. (**12**) ....

example:	**A** **B** **C** **D** **E** **F** **G** **H** **I** ☐ ■ ☐ ☐ ☐ ☐ ☐ ☐ ☐

A Unfortunately, many departments don't want to share their specialist knowledge with others.

B It is this: just as the Internet connects people around the world, intranets connect people within a single company.

C The more information it has, the more people will use it.

D In this way, people can get the information they need, regardless of where it comes from.

E Most employees prefer to communicate by telephone or in writing.

F But an intranet should provide important information which people need to make decisions about new products, costings and so on.

G This means that you do not have to buy a lot of additional programs to set up an intranet service.

H That is, they use the intranet to give orders, not to exchange information between themselves and others working in the same organisation.

I Of course, if they don't have a computer terminal, they cannot make use of the system.

PART THREE

Questions 13–20

- Read this text about the People's Bank of Sri Lanka.
- Answer questions **13–20** on the opposite page.

The People's Bank

The People's Bank is one of Sri Lanka's biggest banks with 6.5 million accounts out of a population of 18.3 million. It provides a full range of domestic and international banking services. In particular, it tries to help the weaker sectors of the economy by providing financing and credit. So far, most of the Bank's branches have been situated in the towns.

1.   But now, one of the main objectives of the People's Bank is to improve financial services throughout the whole country. To achieve this goal, the Bank has taken a number of measures, including: opening branches in rural areas, recruiting staff locally and carrying out business dealings in local languages. Above all, it has created a new village-based institution called the 'Rural Bank'.

2.   There are now 1,206 Rural Banks countrywide, with more planned. The People's Bank has identified the needs of the rural sector and has introduced various credit schemes to suit farmers and other rural entrepreneurs. For example, the bank has granted credit for rice cultivation. It is also providing credit facilities to the organisations which buy agricultural produce from farmers. In this way, farmers can sell their crops during the harvesting seasons instead of having to wait or store them.

3.   The People's Bank understands the importance of the Micro Small and Medium Enterprise (MSME) sector in creating employment and encouraging economic activity. Unlike large factory-based centralised enterprises, which go in for mass production of a few products, the small and medium enterprises in the MSME sector cover a wide range of products. A good example of the way in which the People's Bank is assisting industrial development in rural areas is its support for electrification: it has already provided more than Rs 2 billion.

4.   The MSME sector is the fastest-growing sector of the Sri Lankan economy. It is clear, too, that small entrepreneurs are desperate for credit facilities. They are already paying very high interest rates to private lenders. The People's Bank intends to provide credit to these small businesses at attractive rates of interest. The People's Bank is therefore working on a scheme aimed specifically at them. It is called the 'Rural Banking Innovation Project', which will be introduced within the next eighteen months. It will have a number of financial innovations, including competitive interest rates, linking credit with savings, and repayment of loans in regular instalments.

Questions 13–16

- For questions **13–16**, choose from the list **A–G** the best title for each numbered paragraph in the text.
- For each numbered paragraph **1–4**, mark **one** letter **A–G** on your Answer Sheet.
- Do not use any letter more than once.

13 Paragraph 1 ....

14 Paragraph 2 ....

15 Paragraph 3 ....

16 Paragraph 4 ....

> **A** Plans for the future
> **B** Urban financial services
> **C** A new kind of bank
> **D** Mass-production and other factory schemes
> **E** Helping agriculture
> **F** Fixing market interest rates
> **G** The importance of investment in rural industries

Questions 17–20

- Using the information in the text, complete each sentence **17–20** with a phrase **A–G** from the list below.
- For each sentence **17–20**, mark **one** letter **A–G** on your Answer Sheet.
- Do not use any letter more than once.

17 Credit facilities for farmers have been introduced to ....

18 A characteristic of small-scale rural industries is that they ....

19 Small businesses need to be able to ....

20 The Rural Bank's policy is to recruit local staff and to ....

> **A** operate in local languages
> **B** increase salaries and other benefits
> **C** borrow money at reasonable rates of interest
> **D** specialise in factory mass production
> **E** make it easier to sell agricultural produce at harvest time
> **F** make more money for the government
> **G** cover many different kinds of products

PART FOUR

Questions 21–35

- Read this report on energy consumption in New Zealand offices.
- Choose the correct word from **A, B, C** or **D** on the opposite page to fill in each gap.
- For each question **21–35**, mark **one** letter **A, B, C** or **D** on your Answer Sheet.

Saving energy in the office

The amount of energy consumed – and wasted – in commercial buildings in New Zealand is increasing all the time. The **(example)** .... in numbers of items of electronic office equipment threatens to reach its maximum in New Zealand's main business centres in the next ten years. Office staff leave equipment **(21)** .... on unnecessarily for a number of reasons. These include fear of **(22)** .... the machine, **(23)** .... of knowledge of the actual cost of running the machine, and just plain laziness.

(24) .... to control the energy usage of office equipment is wasteful, and can **(25)** .... to costs far higher than most managers **(26)** .... The Energy Efficiency & **(27)** .... Authority (EECA) is introducing a twofold programme aimed at **(28)** .... the $50m which is wasted every year in New Zealand's offices. Office machines in New Zealand consume 370 GWh of energy per year, or about 1% of the country's **(29)** .... electricity consumption.

Further, the EECA now **(30)** .... that the number of office machines will double before the end of the decade. By this time, office machinery energy consumption is **(31)** .... to be about 800 gW per year.

A recent EECA survey of offices in the capital city's central business **(32)** .... revealed that 40% of office equipment was left **(33)** .... overnight and through the weekend, as well as in working hours. It also found that about half the energy consumed during office hours is wasted, because machines remain on when not in **(34)** .... In particular, most PCs, printers and photocopiers are fully **(35)** .... for only about 40% of a working day.

Example:

A growth   B count   C progress   D result

example:	A B C D
	■ □ □ □

21	A	driven	B	switched	C	remained	D	stayed
22	A	hurting	B	offending	C	damaging	D	spoiling
23	A	lack	B	need	C	want	D	gap
24	A	Neglect	B	Prevention	C	Loss	D	Failure
25	A	come	B	take	C	keep	D	lead
26	A	decide	B	realise	C	explain	D	produce
27	A	Conservation	B	Contract	C	Convert	D	Conference
28	A	sparing	B	controlling	C	saving	D	removing
29	A	same	B	whole	C	total	D	all
30	A	estimates	B	proposes	C	foretells	D	guesses
31	A	told	B	expected	C	awaited	D	argued
32	A	environment	B	district	C	region	D	section
33	A	circulating	B	going	C	playing	D	running
34	A	place	B	work	C	use	D	time
35	A	exercised	B	operated	C	handled	D	utilised

PART FIVE

Section A

Questions 36–40

- Read this news item about an agreement between Australia and Japan.
- In most of the lines **36–40** there is **one extra word** which does not fit. One or two lines, however, are correct.
- If a line is correct, put a tick (✔) in the space on your Answer Sheet.
- If there is an extra word in the line, write that word in the space on your Answer Sheet.

Examples:

We should like to apologise for the delay, and can assure you that .... ✔ ....

such as a thing will not happen again. .... *as* ....

　　　The Australian Wheat Board, the centralised export marketing agency, said

36　yesterday that it had been signed a A$400m agreement with Japan covering

37　at least 900,000 tonnes of wheat for the coming year. Japanese customers

38　have agreed with to take 660,000 tonnes of Australian Standard White wheat,

39　which is used mainly for the making Udon noodles, and 240,000 tonnes of

40　Prime Hard Wheat. Japan, which one of the largest customers for Australian

　　　wheat, has taken around 1m tonnes annually for the past decade.

PART FIVE

Section B

Questions 41–45

- A colleague of yours has written a memo and has asked you to check it.
- In each line there is **one wrong word**.
- For each line **41–45**, write the **correct word** in the space on your Answer Sheet.

Examples:

When you application for a job, always send a covering letter with your CV. .... *apply* ....

Your letter should be neat written. .... *neatly* ....

Damage to paper shredders from paper clips and staples

Please remove staples and paper clips from documents before shredding

41   them. The finer the cut that a paper shredder makes, the more likelihood

42   it is to suffer damaged from paper clips and staples. A large strip cut

43   shredder will 'eat' paper clips and staples for years without causing no

44   noticeable damage. On the other's hand, the fine particle cut shredder

45   which we use to destroy confidential documents can easy be damaged

  by a single staple. So, please take care!

WRITING

Questions 46 and 47

PART ONE

Question 46

- You are the Manager of a Motor Insurance office. You are concerned about the size of recent telephone bills. You suspect that staff talk too much on the phone, and that some are using the phones for personal use.
- Write a memo of **30–40 words** to all members of staff about the problem, including:
  - costs
  - the length of phone calls
  - personal use of office phones.
- **Write on your Answer Sheet.**

PART TWO

Question 47

- You are the Purchasing Officer for Freeman Process Engineering, and you have received a communication from Better Business Systems confirming your order for new office furniture.

1   Confirmation of order from BBS.

Better Business Systems

OFFICE FITTING AND REFURBISHING

Confirmation of order

To: Purchasing Officer, Freeman Process Engineering

From: James Carter, Sales

Date: 2 July 1999

Re: Order no. 345678

Further to our telephone conversation, I confirm the following arrangements for supply and delivery of assorted office furniture to your new offices in Cardiff.

Office furniture required:

Item	Description	Colour	Quantity
DESK	1500 x 750 with 3 drawers	grey melamine	2
BOOKCASE	1800 x 900 with 5 adjustable shelves	grey melamine	2
CHAIR	Clerical/typist with arms. Fabric: wool	red	6
FILING CABINET	4-drawer, steel	grey	3

Delivery date

30 November 1999

Lighting and flooring

As agreed, our consultant will meet your Managing Director on site next Friday, 13 July at 10.30 to discuss your requirements.

Better Business Systems

BBS House
Dawley Business Park
Telford TF34 3JJ
Tel: 01952 275185

- Your Managing Director has read the BBS confirmation of order, and has sent you a memo about it.

2   Memo from your Managing Director

To: Purchasing Officer

From: Managing Director

Date: 5 July 1999

Re: Your order to BBS for new office furniture

Thank you for attending to this matter so promptly. Unfortunately, one or two changes are needed. Please get in touch with BBS and make the following amendments:

1   I don't like grey. Change to beige, at least for the desk and bookcase.

2   I assume the typists' chairs with arms are more expensive. If so, get chairs without arms.

3   I suggest you order four not three filing cabinets.

4   The delivery date is satisfactory, but they must deliver in the morning.

Re the site meeting, I cannot manage that date after all. Get Carter's secretary to phone mine to fix a new date.

- Write a letter of **100–120 words** to BBS asking for the changes your Managing Director wants. Use the information in the confirmation of order and the memo above.
- You are advised to lay out your letter properly. The words in the address will not count in the 120 word limit.
- **Write on your Answer Sheet**.

LISTENING   Approximately 40 minutes (including 10 minutes transfer time)

PART ONE

Questions 1–12

- You will hear three telephone conversations.
- Write **one** or **two** words in the numbered spaces on the forms below.
- After each conversation, rewind the tape and listen again.

Conversation One
(Questions 1–4)

- Look at the form below.
- You will hear a woman talking to an employment agency.

PERSONPLAN EMPLOYMENT AGENCY

Date and time of message: 12/5/98   4.30 p.m.

Caller: Janet Cross
Name of Company: Universal Lift Inc.
Staff required: **(1)** ....
Skills required: **(2)** .... **(3)** ....
To start work: **(4)** ....

Contact number: (212) 465 7023

Conversation Two
(Questions 5–8)

- Look at the form below.
- You will hear a man talking to a catering services department.

Catering Services Department
Message

To: Victoria Evans
Date: 7/9/98
Time: 10.30 a.m.

Mr Moss from **(5)** .... division rang. He wants to order a dinner on **(6)** .... for 15. He wants it served in the **(7)** .... dining room with at least three **(8)** ....

Can you get back to him as soon as possible?

37

**Conversation Three
(Questions 9–12)**

- Look at the diary below.
- You will hear two people discussing appointments.

September 1998   Week 38

- -

16 Monday
9.30 meeting with **(9)** ....
(10) .... with Lee Van Canh

_____

17 Tuesday
Visit **(11)** .... (all day)

_____

18 Wednesday
2.15 p.m. **(12)** ....

PART TWO

Questions 13–22

**Section One
(Questions 13–17)**

- You will hear five short advertisements.
- For each piece, decide which topic **A–H** the speaker is talking about.
- Write **one** letter **A–H** next to the number of the piece.
- Do not use any letter more than once.
- At the end of question 17, rewind the tape and listen again.

13 ....

14 ....

15 ....

16 ....

17 ....

A promotional packages
B training courses
C conference venues
D web site designers
E after-dinner speakers
F transportation systems
G pension schemes
H security systems

Section Two
(Questions 18–22)

- You will hear five speakers talking about different departments of an organisation.
- For each piece, decide which department **A–H** the speaker is talking about.
- Write **one** letter **A–H** next to the number of the piece.
- Do not use any letter more than once.
- At the end of question 22, rewind the tape and listen again.

18 ....

19 ....

20 ....

21 ....

22 ....

A research & development
B information technology
C human resources
D payroll
E publicity
F reception
G shop floor
H canteen

PART THREE

Questions 23–30

- You will hear an interview with Carol Vogel, the President of Telekom. She is talking about their current situation and future prospects.
- Choose the best phrase to answer or complete questions **23–30**.
- Mark **one** letter **A**, **B** or **C** for the answer you choose.
- At the end of the interview, rewind the tape and listen again.

23 What effect will the current financial situation have on Telekom?

    A   It will reduce short-term investment.
    B   It will have no effect on investment.
    C   It will increase long-term investment.

24 What has happened to some of Telekom's projects?

    A   They have been put out to foreign tender.
    B   They have been cancelled.
    C   They have been postponed.

25 What unique situation does Telekom have to face?

    A   The country has very low GDP.
    B   The country is made up of many islands.
    C   The country is densely populated.

26 How many lines per hundred people are Telekom hoping to install?

    A   3
    B   5
    C   60

27 What correct decision does she think the government made?

    A   to privatise the system
    B   to encourage foreign investors
    C   to cooperate with other countries in the region

28 What will international groups do in 15 years' time?

    A   hand back the lines to Telekom
    B   claim back their initial investment
    C   renew their contracts with Telekom

29 Who owns the mobile communications operations?

    A   the government
    B   Telekom
    C   suppliers in a joint venture with Telekom

30 How does the President feel about the future of Telekom?

    A   She is confident it will succeed.
    B   She feels worried things will go wrong.
    C   She has no idea what will happen.

> **You now have 10 minutes to transfer your answers
> to your Answer Sheet.**

SPEAKING   Approximately 18 minutes

Business seminars
*For **three** candidates*

Candidate A

YOUR QUESTIONS

In this activity you will exchange information with your partners about business seminars. You will then discuss with your partners which one you prefer to attend. First find out more about the Financial Accounting seminar. Ask candidate B your questions.

1 Location: ....

2 Focus: ....

3 Date and time: ....

Discussion:

Discuss with your partner which seminar is most appropriate for you. Consider the content and any other details you think are important.

INFORMATION

Candidate C will ask you questions about the seminar on International Trading Techniques. Use the information below to answer the questions.

CAGV are organising a seminar on 'International Trade Techniques'

Seminar Objective: to develop a greater understanding of international trading methods
Topics: International purchasing, export techniques, marketing, banking
Participants will be: senior managers in import-export enterprises
Duration: Tuesday 2/11/97 to Saturday 6/12/97 (8.30 – 11.30 a.m. every morning)
Seminar fee: US$100
Language: Vietnamese/English

Please contact: CAGV Tel: 869 12 66 – Fax: 869 15 39

Business seminars
*For **three** candidates*

Candidate B

YOUR QUESTIONS

In this activity you will exchange information with your partners about business seminars. You will then discuss with your partners which seminar is most appropriate for you. First find out more about the Hartingdon Business School seminar. Ask candidate C your questions.

1 Title: ....

2 Aimed at: ....

3 Further details: ....

Discussion:

Discuss with your partners which seminar is most appropriate for you. Consider the content and any other details you think are important.

INFORMATION

Candidate A will ask you questions about the Financial Accounting Seminar. Use the information below to answer the questions.

FINANCIAL ACCOUNTING SEMINAR

* To be conducted in Hanoi at the Daewoo Hotel by an internationally qualified accountant
* Emphasis on international accounting standards
* 19 November 1997
  morning, 09.30 – 12.30, afternoon, 14.30 – 17.30
* For further information and registration details please contact Ms Dung on Tel: (04) 8 234 125 or Fax: (04) 8 234 876

**BURNE GRIFFTHS
(VIETNAM) LTD**
Certified Chartered Accountants and Management Consultants

Business seminars
*For **three** candidates*

Candidate C

YOUR QUESTIONS

In this activity you will exchange information with your partners about business seminars. You will then discuss with your partners which seminar is most appropriate for you. First find out more about the International Trading Techniques seminar. Ask candidate A your questions.

1 Purpose: ....

2 Participants: ....

3 Duration: ....

Discussion:

Discuss with your partners which seminar is most appropriate for you. Consider the content and any other details you think are important.

INFORMATION

Candidate B will ask you questions about the Hartingdon Business School seminar. Use the information below to answer the questions.

Hartingdon Business School

Are you a manager in a small or medium-sized company?
On Tuesday, 27 August there will be

A Full-Day Seminar on: Listening to Customers

We will
- give you the tools to improve profitability
- help you learn how to put customers at the centre of your business
- deal successfully with customer complaints

Phone/Fax John Bennet on 0171 4356 7888 for more details

Test 3

READING AND WRITING   1 hour 30 minutes

READING

Questions 1–45

PART ONE

Questions 1–7

- Read these sentences and the business cards of four different people on the opposite page.
- Which person does each sentence **1–7** refer to?
- For each sentence, mark **one** letter **A**, **B**, **C** or **D** on your Answer Sheet.
- You will need to use some of the letters more than once.

Example:	**Answer**
This person can help you sell something by auction.	■ ☐ ☐ ☐ A B C D

1 Talk to this person if you need advice on financial matters.

2 This person is involved in overseas trade.

3 This person has offices in several cities.

4 You can contact this person by fax or electronic mail.

5 You could phone this person at home.

6 This person knows several foreign languages.

7 We don't know what this person's job title is.

A

Rossman Pantile
Valuers and auctioneers

Liz Read

Pindar House Castle Place Tinmouth Street London SE11 7HH
Tel   0171 963 3596   Fax   0171 963 3535   e-mail   read@ross.demon.co.uk

B

Private telephone: 01708 997826

Bill Sheppey
Export Manager

Naughton Webster   Thorneycliffe Chesterton
Precision   Sheffield S50 4PP
Engineering   Tel 01742 346180
Limited   Fax 01742 346181

C

Pallo Marson Huazhen   *Certified Public Accountants*
Li Tong Senior Consultant Economist
Suite 6969   Zone 2 Yanze   Room 721
Yu Quan Centre   Wyatt Hotel   410 Huan Shi Rd W
Hua Jia Lou   2222 Yanan Xi Rd   Guangzhou
Beijing   Shanghai 200355   China 5110070
Tel 86 1 422023   Tel 275 4998   Tel 335 0771
Fax 86 1 422422   Fax 275 5000   Tlx 74321

D

Anadolu Translation Agency
Ayşen Ömer-Johnson, MA, Member of the Society of Linguists
Director, Interpreters' Division

Soğuk Su Sokak 19/5
Ankara
Turkey   Tel +90 312 277 4350   Fax +90 312 277 4377

PART TWO

Questions 8–12

- Read this text about the paperless office.
- Choose the best sentence from the opposite page to fill in each of the gaps.
- For each gap **8–12**, mark one letter **A–I** on your Answer Sheet.
- Do not use any letter more than once.

Despite advances in data-storage technology, huge hard-disk drives and computer faxes, the volume of paper in the average office has continued to grow. **(example)** ....

While the younger generation are comfortable working on screen, a lot of older people are not happy with a document draft unless they have a printed copy of it. **(8)** ....

Older computer programs were generally not capable of producing screen previews of what was to be printed, and you simply had to see a draft copy. **(9)** ....

This led to more copies, until the computer software finally produced a satisfactory document. **(10)** ....

Word processing programs today are capable of showing, on screen, exactly what the output will look like, so that hard-copy drafts are generally not required for documents, spreadsheets, etc. **(11)** ....

But, in doing so, they miss the point, because the document is already on file. **(12)** ....

On the other hand, disk drives are now big and cheap enough that they are a much better way of storing data.

---

example:	A	B	C	D	E	F	G	H	I
	☐	☐	☐	☐	☐	☐	■	☐	☐

A Those days are now long gone.

B Printing it out is wasteful, because laser cartridges and paper are both very expensive.

C Of course, you need to know exactly where everything is filed so you can easily find it again.

D There used to be a good reason for this.

E Consider, for example, how much time it takes to send a fax.

F This draft would then need to be corrected for layout several times.

G The reason for this is computers with printers.

H It may be that the final copy needs to be on paper, but the first five drafts should not be.

I But, even though they don't need to print out documents any more, people still want copies 'for the file'.

PART THREE

Questions 13–20

- Read this text about doing business in Brazil.
- Answer questions **13–20** on the opposite page.

Doing business in Brazil

Brazilians take pride in their Portuguese heritage, so to call locals Spanish Americans would be insulting. On the same note, Brazil's official language is Portuguese, not Spanish. Frequently, the spelling of Portuguese words is exactly the same as Spanish, but the pronunciation differs greatly. Before opening your mouth in this country, learn to speak a few words and avoid committing a cultural offence.

1. If your business destination is one of the northern cities like Rio, city of carnival and the samba, expect a somewhat casual environment. However, when scheduling meetings in southern cities, you'll find business settings just the opposite: quite formal. Bring comfortable semi-casual clothes for business in the north, and conservative dark suits or dresses for southern cities like São Paolo.

2. Time is important to southerners and lateness is considered rude and unbusinesslike. In the north, however, your host may not always be so punctual. If you called a meeting at four, a Rio citizen, for example, may interpret gathering time as around four (like maybe four fifteen or so). Whatever you do, don't be put off or indicate that you were concerned about the late arrival; your South American counterpart won't understand.

3. Shaking hands and exchanging business cards begin any first business meeting in Brazil. At that time, introductions are made. Formalise your contact's first name by preceding it with *Senhor, Senhora* or *Senhorita* (Mr, Mrs or Miss). The surname is not generally used. Soon after this formality, the title is usually dropped at the request of your host. Once you've become friendly with *Senhora* Astrud, you would be expected to simply call her Astrud.

4. If you are indicating approval on a business matter, never give the okay sign of a ring formed by the thumb and index finger. This is an obscene gesture in Brazil. Instead, close the fist and shoot the thumb up. During the business day you will most likely be offered *cafezinho*, a very strong Brazilian coffee. Accept it graciously so as not to offend your host. If you don't like coffee, sip it slowly. People from the United States should never refer to their country as 'America'. It is better to say you're from the United States. South Americans, particularly Brazilians, find North Americans a bit egocentric when referring to back home as 'America'. After all, Brazilians live in America too.

Questions 13–16

- For questions **13–16**, choose from the list **A–G** the best title for each numbered paragraph in the text.
- For each numbered paragraph **1–4**, mark **one** letter **A–G** on your Answer Sheet.
- Do not use any letter more than once.

13 Paragraph 1 ....

14 Paragraph 2 ....

15 Paragraph 3 ....

16 Paragraph 4 ....

A Some important business customs
B Advice on speaking the language
C Advice on dress
D Where to do business in Brazil
E Some things to avoid
F Some American habits
G Advice on punctuality

Questions 17–20

- Using the information in the text, complete each sentence **17–20** with a phrase **A–G** from the list below.
- For each sentence **17–20**, mark **one** letter **A–G** on your Answer Sheet.
- Do not use any letter more than once.

17 You should not refer to Spanish Americans because ....

18 You should take two different kinds of clothing to Brazil because ....

19 The rule about using the first names of your business contacts is that ....

20 The problem with using gestures is that ....

A you can easily offend people if you use the wrong one
B São Paolo and Rio have different customs in this respect
C US citizens are also Americans
D they may be offended if you refuse
E you must wait until the Brazilians ask you to do so
F it is customary to hand out business cards first
G Brazil is proud of its Portuguese heritage

PART FOUR

Questions 21–35

- Read this article about a new fund in India.
- Choose the correct word or words from **A, B, C** or **D** on the opposite page to fill in each gap.
- For each question **21–35**, mark **one** letter **A, B, C** or **D** on your Answer Sheet.

Edible oil prices

Navinbhai Shah, President of the Bombay Oilseeds and Oil Exchange, reported this week that edible oil prices have remained high in India throughout the summer. **(example)** .... Mr Shah, this is because a number of festivals such as Dussehra and Diwali are taking place and the **(21)** .... for edible oils is always at its greatest at this time. Shah predicts, however, that prices are **(22)** .... to fall next month when the new oilseed crop starts arriving.

Traders said palm oil was **(23)** .... at Rs 27,000 a tonne in the domestic markets, while groundnut oil fetched the higher price of Rs 35,000 a tonne. Industry officials said domestic edible oil prices had also **(24)** .... in line with Malaysian palm oil prices. Malaysian prices have gone up because it seems that *El Niño* had **(25)** .... the oilseed crop in some parts.

El Niño is a weather phenomenon that **(26)** .... a rise in sea surface temperatures in the eastern Pacific and a cooling in the western Pacific around Southeast Asia. The change can disrupt weather **(27)** .... worldwide, leading to drought in Indonesia and Australia and floods in South America. The present *El Niño* that is developing is believed to be one of the strongest **(28)** .... Trade officials said that more imported oils than **(29)** .... were arriving at Indian ports, because of the festivals and the end of the domestic **(30)** ....

The new oilseed **(31)** .... normally starts arriving from late October, and imports start to come down from November as domestic **(32)** .... increase. The government **(33)** .... that the 1997–98 (July–June) winter oilseed output will be about 13.46 million tonnes **(34)** .... with more than 14 million tonnes in 1996–97.

The country harvests two oilseed crops, and receives the **(35)** .... of its output from the winter crop.

Example:

A According to   B Except for   C Because of   D Taking after

example:	**A**	**B**	**C**	**D**
	▄	☐	☐	☐

		A		B		C		D	
21	**A**	enquiry	**B**	demand	**C**	request	**D**	order
22	**A**	able	**B**	seen	**C**	known	**D**	likely
23	**A**	stated	**B**	told	**C**	repeated	**D**	quoted
24	**A**	risen	**B**	burst	**C**	expanded	**D**	gained
25	**A**	broken	**B**	injured	**C**	managed	**D**	affected
26	**A**	causes	**B**	does	**C**	makes	**D**	sends
27	**A**	maps	**B**	forecasts	**C**	patterns	**D**	storms
28	**A**	by heart	**B**	on record	**C**	in time	**D**	from memory
29	**A**	once	**B**	always	**C**	now	**D**	usual
30	**A**	duration	**B**	season	**C**	period	**D**	stage
31	**A**	freight	**B**	plant	**C**	crop	**D**	surplus
32	**A**	records	**B**	numbers	**C**	supplies	**D**	issues
33	**A**	intends	**B**	calculates	**C**	values	**D**	recommends
34	**A**	confronted	**B**	measured	**C**	compared	**D**	assessed
35	**A**	bulk	**B**	share	**C**	weight	**D**	part

PART FIVE

Section A

Questions 36–40

- Read this note on recycling office paper.
- In most of the lines **36–40** there is **one extra word** which does not fit. One or two lines, however, are correct.
- If a line is correct, put a tick (✔) in the space on your Answer Sheet.
- If there is an extra word in the line, write that word in the space on your Answer Sheet.

Examples:

We should like to apologise for the delay, and can assure you that   .... ✔ ....

such as a thing will not happen again.   .... *as* ....

Recycling office paper is important because it reduces the demand for

36   paper made from new wood-pulp, and therefore the need of to plant new

37   forests. It also reduces the amount of energy needed for processing new

38   wood-pulp. Not all paper can it be recycled, so there should be two

39   separate bins in each office. One bin is for recyclable paper like as

40   computer printout paper and office stationery. The one other is for paper

which makes poor quality recycled paper, e.g. card and glossy magazines.

PART FIVE

Section B

Questions 41–45

- A colleague of yours has written a memo and has asked you to check it.
- In each line there is **one wrong word**.
- For each line **41–45**, write the **correct word** in the space on your Answer Sheet.

Examples:

When you application for a job, always send a covering letter with your CV. .... *apply* ....

Your letter should be neat written. .... *neatly* ....

Visas

Tourists can enter Sri Lanka without a visa. They may remain for

41 90 days without payment. Foreigners coming for businesses

42 purposes can stay for up to 30 days. Any period in exceed of

43 three months incur a temporary residence tax of Rs 2,500. If

44 you entry on a tourist visa, you cannot change its status. There

45 is also a scheme under which professionals who's expertise is

not available here can obtain a 5-year resident visa.

WRITING

Questions 46 and 47

PART ONE

Question 46

- You are the Chief Accountant for an Import-Export Agency. You have seen an advertisement for a short training course about a new financial management program.
- Write a memo of **30–40 words** to your boss to include:
    - a request to go on the course
    - some details about the course (e.g. date, cost)
    - why you think the course will be useful.
- **Write on your Answer Sheet.**

PART TWO

Question 47

- You are assistant to the Office Manager. Your company is planning to move office, and you have received a memo from your boss.

1   Memo from Office Manager

Re: Moving office from Cambridge to Bristol

Get in touch with Mrs Morton of Flash removals to find out the following: costs for removal; storage of items not wanted immediately; handling of our fragile laboratory equipment; cost to us if they do the packing for us; insurance costs. Also, check if a moving date in mid-May is acceptable to them. I suggest you ask them to visit us here in Cambridge to work out an estimate of total costs.

JSB
Office Manager

- You have received a reply from Flash removals and sent it to your Office Manager. You make some notes of the phone call from your Office Manager after he has read the reply from Flash Removals.

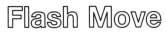

Flash Move
INTERNATIONAL
COMMERCIAL REMOVALS

Office and laboratory
Haulage and Storage
Full packing service
Factory and warehouse
Hi-tech removals   *National and International*
Full loads and single items   *Professional planning advice*
Document storage   *Careful and helpful uniformed porters*
Crate hire

Full insurance cover – 24 hr service
Free survey and estimates – Surprisingly low rates

                                Cambridge 01223 908001
Member of   24 hour mobile 0891 187666
Freight Transport   Head office: Carter House, Lade Way,
Association   Cambridge CB9 1EE

---

2   Your notes of the phone call

Removal costs	no problem
Date	check if change to Oct OK
Cost of packing	query this – includes fragile equipment?
Insurance	what does this cover?
Storage	too expensive – sell old furniture instead
Flash visit	the date they suggest not convenient – re-arrange

- Write a letter of **100–120 words** to Mrs Morton dealing with the points made by your boss. Use the information above.
- You are advised to lay out your letter properly. The words in the address will not count in the 120 word limit.
- **Write on your Answer Sheet.**

LISTENING   Approximately 40 minutes (including 10 minutes transfer time)

PART ONE

Questions 1–12

- You will hear three telephone conversations.
- Write **one** or **two** words or a number in the numbered spaces on the forms below.
- After each conversation, rewind the tape and listen again.

Conversation One
(Questions 1–4)

- Look at the form below.
- A woman is leaving instructions for her assistant.

Tuesday, 5 November

<u>Tasks</u>

1.   Ask **(1)** .... to network computers in the Marketing Division.
      Then **(2)** .... Group.

2.   Make appointment with James on **(3)** .... at .... a.m.

3.   Book **(4)** .... for this evening

---

Conversation Two
(Questions 5–8)

- Look at the form below.
- You will hear a man complaining to his bank.

12/5/99

Customer Name: Frank Bailey

(5) .... : 5220 4768

- ◆ **(6)** .... (£2,000) has been paid into deposit rather than current account, customer is now **(7)** ....: letter sent to customer and charge made.
- ◆ customer reports unauthorised withdrawals of **(8)** .... from account
- ◆ customer's cash-point card rejected

Conversation Three
(Questions 9–12)

- Look at the form below.
- You will hear a woman talking about flight arrangements.

Memo

To: Ann Burton
From: Travel Desk
Subject: Flights for your visit to the Philippines

Flights out:
BA 027 at 21.30 arrives **(9)** .... at 17.40
KLM 221 at 19.10 to Manila*

*Very **(10)** .... transfer time

or

BA 171 at 15.00 to Amsterdam followed by CP333 to Manila**

flight is full but you could be wait-listed; also there's a **(11) .... wait at Amsterdam!

Flights back:
CP 908 Manila-London, only **(12)** .... seat available (same fare)

PART TWO

Questions 13–22

Section One
(Questions 13–17)

- You will hear five people talking in different places.
- For each piece, choose the location **A–H** where the person is speaking.
- Write **one** letter **A–H** next to the number of the piece.
- Do not use any letter more than once.
- After question 17, rewind the tape and listen again.

13 ....

14 ....

15 ....

16 ....

17 ....

A	office
B	hospital
C	factory
D	airport
E	bank
F	shop
G	hotel
H	car park

Section Two
(Questions 18–22)

- You will hear five people talking on the phone.
- For each piece, decide the reason **A–H** for the telephone call.
- Write **one** letter **A–H** next to the number of the piece.
- Do not use any letter more than once.
- At the end of question 22, rewind the tape and listen again.

18 ....

19 ....

20 ....

21 ....

22 ....

A	make an appointment
B	check an address
C	congratulate someone
D	offer a lift
E	sell something
F	place an order
G	cancel a meeting
H	book a table

PART THREE

Questions 23–30

- You will hear Paul talk about how he set up his own business to advise companies about their information technology needs.
- Choose the best phrase to answer or complete questions **23–30**.
- Mark **one** letter **A**, **B** or **C** for the answer you choose.
- At the end of the talk, rewind the tape and listen again.

23 What does Paul think is dangerous for businesses?

    A   lack of IT knowledge
    B   not using the Internet
    C   hiding their problems

24 What aspects of his company is Paul proud of?

    A   It is long-established.
    B   It provides a comprehensive service.
    C   It has a proven record of success.

25 What does Paul's company offer?

    A   high-quality hardware
    B   tailor-made software
    C   technical assistance

26 Why did his first company fail?

    A   lack of investment in the business
    B   staff demands that couldn't be met
    C   disagreements between the partners

27 What has he done to make sure his new company is successful?

    A   He remains the sole owner.
    B   He is keeping it small.
    C   He does not take risks.

28 His staff like working for him because

    A   they are paid well.
    B   they find it an exciting place to work.
    C   they are involved in making decisions.

29 What does he find most satisfying about his work?

    A   He can live where he wants.
    B   He has made a lot of money.
    C   He knows what he wants to do.

30 What does he want to do in the future?

    A   sell the company
    B   retire to the country
    C   start a new business

**You now have 10 minutes to transfer your answers
to your Answer Sheet.**

SPEAKING   Approximately 12 minutes

Removals and storage
*For **two** candidates*

Candidate A

YOUR QUESTIONS

In this activity you will find out information about two companies which specialise
in international removal and storage services. You will then discuss with your
partner which one you would prefer to use. First find out more about ACE
Removals. Ask candidate B your questions.

---

1 Specialist services: ....

2 Established: ....

3 Countries: ....

Discussion:

Discuss with your partner which removal and storage service you would prefer to use.
Consider the range of services offered and any other details you think are important.

INFORMATION

Your partner will ask you questions about International Movers. Use the
information below to answer the questions.

INTERNATIONAL MOVERS CO. LTD.

◆ Door to door moving service by sea or air freight
◆ Professional export packing service using international standard packing
  materials
◆ Professionally trained packers
◆ Apartment/villa and office moving
◆ Import customs clearance
◆ 24 hour security warehousing facility
◆ Offices in over 40 countries worldwide

Tel: 885 3069
Mobile phone: 0 908 0 9393

Removals and storage
*For **two** candidates*

Candidate B

In this activity you will find out information about two companies who specialise in international removal and storage services. You will then discuss with your partner which one you would prefer to use. First find out more about International Movers Co. Ltd. Ask candidate A your questions.

1 Packers:	....
2 Customs service:	....
3 Branches:	....

Discussion:

Discuss with your partner which removal and storage service you would prefer to use. Consider the range of services offered and any other details you think are important.

INFORMATION

Your partner will ask you questions about ACE Removals. Use the information below to answer the questions.

ACE REMOVALS

Specialist packers and shippers of personal effects, antiques, fine art and motor vehicles

Experience in USA, AUSTRALIA, NEW ZEALAND, CANADA, SOUTH AFRICA & FAR EAST

Immediate Quotations – 7 Days a Week

01223 32888222

Head Office: A1 Radford Business Centre, Billericay, Essex CM12 0BZ

Test 4

READING AND WRITING   1 hour 30 minutes

READING

Questions 1–45

PART ONE

Questions 1–7

- Look at the sentences below and the conference notices on page 64.
- Which event does each sentence **1–7** refer to?
- For each sentence, mark **one** letter **A**, **B**, **C** or **D** on your Answer Sheet.
- You will need to use some of the letters more than once.

Example:	Answer
You should book early for this event.	A☐ B☐ C■ D☐

1 This event is of particular interest to people who work in financial institutions.

2 You will have to share a room if you attend this event.

3 This is the place to learn about organising conference events.

4 If you want to learn how to get on in your career, go to this event.

5 There is no charge for this event.

6 If your job involves documents in foreign languages, this event will interest you.

7 This event will be useful if you have a number of people working under you.

A

The **Business Communicator Conference** is designed for all Personal Assistants and Private Secretaries who want to improve their presentation skills, gain added confidence through assertiveness training and learn a whole host of business information. It is an opportunity for you to 'network' with other people in your profession. Conference fees include accommodation in twin-bedded bedrooms, all meals and transfer to and from the conference centre.

B

The **Senior Secretarial Congress** offers an opportunity for Executive Secretaries to keep abreast of developments in their field, to gain an insight into the changes influencing their roles, and above all to demonstrate ways of developing their careers. The key issues to be covered include: dealing with change, managing staff, communication skills and personal career planning. The cost of the 2-day conference includes all course notes, refreshments and lunch.

C

The **Executive Secretary Show** provides an opportunity to broaden your business contacts and to gain practical advice from experts in such key areas as office products, business technology, organising conferences, incentive travel and corporate hospitality. Experts will also be on hand to advise on effective purchasing practices and ways in which to increase the efficiency of your office. Admission is free, but you are advised to book early as places are limited.

D

The **PA Specialist Forum** is of particular interest to senior secretarial staff working in specialist areas, including banking, accountancy, stockbroking and financial services. Seminar topics include technical report writing, translation from and into other languages and presenting statistical information. There will also be workshops in specific computer-related areas, including graphics packages and the use of spreadsheets and databases. Please note that the fee covers all seminars, one workshop and all course materials.

PART TWO

Questions 8–12

- Read this text about business opportunities in Vietnam.
- Choose the best sentence from page 66 to fill in each of the gaps.
- For each gap **8–12**, mark one letter **A–I** on your Answer Sheet.
- Do not use any letter more than once.

Business opportunities in Vietnam

Business opportunities in Vietnam are enormous. The rate of growth here is among the highest in the world. (**example**) ....

Vietnam is well-placed for economic development, because it is part of ASEAN. (**8**) ....

It is fortunate, too, to be surrounded by countries with large populations, e.g. China, Laos, Cambodia, Myanmar and Thailand. (**9**) ....

The opportunities for business abound, but remember that the first are always rewarded with the best chances of getting quality business contacts. (**10**) ....

So, the best thing to do to start with is to select contacts with companies similar to your own, and companies which you consider could be interested in your line of products or services. (**11**) ....

In the letter, present yourself and the products you deal with in a clear and simple manner. (**12**) ....

The chances of getting a reply are more than if you had used other types of communication.

---

example:	A B C D E F G H I ☐ ☐ ☐ ☐ ☐ ☐ ■ ☐ ☐

A All of these offer large markets for any product produced in Vietnam.

B A large number of them are small, privately owned companies.

C The next thing is to write a letter (no fax, e-mail or phone calls).

D This means that it can reach customers not only in Indo-China but in the other ASEAN nations.

E It boasts a strong, young labour force of 36 million and a literacy rate of 88%.

F The first impression may be the last impression so you must be very precise and very specific.

G It reaches all sectors of the economy and is likely to accelerate in the future.

H Vietnam's industry could be somewhat like that of Taiwan in a few years' time.

I Remember, too, that business is best done through human contact, not by machines.

PART THREE

Questions 13–20

- Read this text about people who start their own business.
- Answer questions **13–20** on page 68.

Starting your own company

What makes managers give up their high salary, company car and pension, and risk everything in order to set up on their own? A recent UK survey of self-employed entrepreneurs has come up with a number of reasons.

1. Although money is a great motivator, it is only part of the answer. Very few self-employed entrepreneurs can earn what they received in a large company, at least in the first few years. They invest any extra cash in their business, rather than in expensive cars, houses or holidays. Probably the most important part of the answer has to do with being in charge. In the US, people who want to make a million don't care whether they own 5% or 10% of the company, but in the UK, entrepreneurs want 100% ownership: they want to *control* their company and to make all the decisions themselves.

2. Most large companies do not know how to make the best use of clever people. Employees who criticise the old ways of doing things and want to try out new ideas are disliked both by their colleagues and by their bosses. Comments like 'They wouldn't listen to me' or 'I kept presenting new product ideas, only to hear nothing' are typical of many a manager-turned-entrepreneur. All of this causes frustration, which can quickly lead to boredom. Often, middle managers start to think: 'Only another 30 more years of working my way to retirement.' At this point, they want to find a way out.

3. They need to get away from a job that is no longer attractive. So they decide to set up on their own. But they need something else, too: the challenge of taking risks. They are like people who climb a mountain by the most dangerous route. Entrepreneurial types need to try out new things without knowing whether they will succeed or fail. They also want to prove that they can make it without big company support.

4. As well as motivation, most successful entrepreneurs have a number of personal characteristics in common. The first is self-confidence, the feeling of certainty that you have got the skills, knowledge and energy to build up your own business. There is also stubbornness, the determination to prove to the boss who rejected your ideas that they were good ideas which can be made to work. Possessing this quality means that you won't give up: you *have* to make your ideas work.

Questions 13–16

- For questions **13–16**, choose from the list **A–G** the best title for each numbered paragraph in the text.
- For each numbered paragraph **1–4**, mark **one** letter **A–G** on your Answer Sheet.
- Do not use any letter more than once.

13 Paragraph 1 ....

14 Paragraph 2 ....

15 Paragraph 3 ....

16 Paragraph 4 ....

A Likes and dislikes
B The waste of talent in big companies
C The need to be your own boss
D Important personal qualities
E Making a lot of money
F Taking risks
G Time and hard work

Questions 17–20

- Using the information in the text, complete each sentence **17–20** with a phrase **A–G** from the list below.
- For each sentence **17–20**, mark **one** letter **A–G** on your Answer Sheet.
- Do not use any letter more than once.

17 When entrepreneurs start to make money, they will probably ....

18 Part of the price for starting on your own is that you have to ....

19 If the company you work for doesn't appreciate your ideas, you are likely to ....

20 One reason for starting your own business is to ....

A think up new ways of making money
B put it back into the business
C find a way out
D feel very frustrated
E realise how long it takes to succeed
F give up things like pensions and a company car
G prove to others that you can make a success of it

PART FOUR

Questions 21–35

- Read this article about the effect of the Asian crisis on Latin American countries.
- Choose the correct word from **A**, **B**, **C** or **D** on page 70 to fill in each gap.
- For each question **21–35**, mark **one** letter **A**, **B**, **C** or **D** on your Answer Sheet.

Asian crisis affects Latin American markets

Latin American stocks fell for a second day on Friday in reaction to Asia's currency and stock market crash. There were fears that the Asian crisis could **(example)** .... investors in other emerging markets.

Argentina and Mexico **(21)** .... the highest falls, with their indexes down by 4% by the **(22)** .... of trading on Friday. Brazil's Bovespa index, which on the same day **(23)** .... by far the steepest plunge in the Americas, was down 2.9%.

'What's happening in Hong Kong has been a terrible **(24)** .... to the system,' said Richard Watt, who **(25)** .... 3.5 billion dollars in emerging market investments for BEA Associates in New York. Investors in Brazil were concerned that its economic problems were dangerously **(26)** .... to those that have caused the currency and market plunges in Thailand, Malaysia and other Asian **(27)** ....

'Brazil's economy is far from **(28)** .... ,' said Ian Campbell, chief economist at ABN Amro Bank NV Amsterdam. 'Its current account and fiscal **(29)** .... are large and its currency is overvalued.' 'There's no **(30)** .... in trying to catch a falling knife,' said Jane Heap, Latin American stock strategist at Deutsche Morgan Grenfell. 'There's no room for **(31)** .... in Brazil until the US and Asia get back to normal.'

There were also concerns that foreign investors who specialise in emerging markets could be **(32)** .... to sell their shares in Latin America to **(33)** .... their Asian losses.

'There's a lot of nervousness about whether investors will **(34)** .... their money out of stocks, because of instability in Asia,' said German Guerrero, chief trader at the Chilean brokerage Celfin SA.

Chilean markets were down only **(35)** .... in afternoon trading. The Chile selective stock index fell 0.72% and the Chile general stock index was down 0.64%.

Example:

A   influence   B   cause   C   decide   D   persuade

example:	A B C D
	■ ☐ ☐ ☐

21	**A**	sent	**B**	experienced	**C**	took	**D**	enjoyed
22	**A**	stop	**B**	cancellation	**C**	close	**D**	collapse
23	**A**	urged	**B**	delivered	**C**	recovered	**D**	suffered
24	**A**	shock	**B**	reaction	**C**	block	**D**	attack
25	**A**	directs	**B**	earns	**C**	deals	**D**	manages
26	**A**	identical	**B**	similar	**C**	equal	**D**	related
27	**A**	capitals	**B**	investments	**C**	markets	**D**	indexes
28	**A**	sound	**B**	high	**C**	true	**D**	hope
29	**A**	debts	**B**	deficits	**C**	shortages	**D**	dues
30	**A**	idea	**B**	help	**C**	price	**D**	point
31	**A**	cure	**B**	renewal	**C**	aid	**D**	improvement
32	**A**	promised	**B**	reminded	**C**	offered	**D**	forced
33	**A**	fill	**B**	pay	**C**	cover	**D**	replace
34	**A**	sell	**B**	pull	**C**	put	**D**	rub
35	**A**	slightly	**B**	really	**C**	fairly	**D**	badly

PART FIVE

Section A

Questions 36–40

- Read this short report about education in Argentina.
- In most of the lines **36–40** there is **one extra word** which does not fit. One or two lines, however, are correct.
- If a line is correct, put a tick (✔) in the space on your Answer Sheet.
- If there is an extra word in the line, write that word in the space on your Answer Sheet.

Examples:

We should like to apologise for the delay, and can assure you that   .... ✔ ....

such as a thing will not happen again.   .... *as* ....

	According to Argentina's Education Minister, the country's educational
36	results are ten times better off than those of the United States. When asked
37	as to defend this statement, she gave the following explanation: states in
38	the US invest between 445,000 and 20,000 dollars per pupil, while in Argentina
39	the range is between 550 and 1,200. Comparing any results, she argued that
40	Argentina's its schools are more efficient, because Argentina pays less
	to get the same results.

PART FIVE

Section B

Questions 41–45

- The Officer Manager has written a memo and has asked you to check it.
- In each line there is **one wrong word**.
- For each line **41–45**, write the **correct word** in the space on your Answer Sheet.

Examples:

When you application for a job, always send a covering letter with your CV. ....*apply*.......

Your letter should be neat written. ....*neatly*.......

To all office staff

Sending faxes

In future all faxes must be sent directly from a PC. Under the

41   old system, a fax had to be print. You then took it to the fax

42   machine. Next, you entered the destination number, and during

43   the fax was being sent, it was necessity to wait to collect it, and

44   finally to file it. All this resulted for a waste of time and resources.

45   Note: staff who do not have a modem attaching to their PC can still

      send faxes using the internal network.

WRITING

Questions 46 and 47

PART ONE

Question 46

- Señor Viladomat, an important Spanish client, is coming to your company for a meeting about a new product. You are responsible for making arrangements for his trip.
- Write a fax of **30–40 words** to Señor Viladomat's secretary, saying what arrangements you have made, including:
  - travel (e.g. arrival details, meeting and transfer)
  - accommodation
  - details of the product meeting (e.g. time, venue).
- **Write on your Answer Sheet.**

PART TWO

Question 47

- The President of Brent Pharmaceuticals, Mr Shilling, is visiting the Ankara branch of the company for the annual board meeting. You are secretary to the Managing Director of Brent Ankara and are responsible for making the arrangements. You have produced a draft plan of Mr Shilling's itinerary and programme.

1 Draft plan

Draft Itinerary and Programme for President's visit to Ankara		
Saturday	09.00	Dep. London Heathrow, flight LH 4040
	11.30	Arr. Frankfurt
	13.05	Dep. Frankfurt, flight LH 3822
	17.20	Arr. Ankara airport
Transfer:	to be met at the Airport by company driver	
Accommodation:	Single Executive Room at the Dedeman Hotel	
Sunday		free day
Monday	08.30	Managing Director to collect from hotel
	09.00 – 12.00	Visit to Company laboratories
	12.00 – 13.30	Lunch at Mangal restaurant
	14.00 – 17.30	Board Meeting
	Evening	Dinner at MD's home
Tuesday	Morning	(to be arranged)
	16.00	Transfer to airport
	18.05	Dep. Ankara, flight LH 4010
	20.35	Arr. Frankfurt
	21.05	Dep. Frankfurt, flight LH 3833
	22.00	Arr. London Heathrow

- You receive a fax from the President's secretary commenting on your draft.

2   Fax

Brent Pharmaceuticals
Poole House
Bridge Street SE23 5RT
Fax 0181 333 3333

FACSIMILE MESSAGE

From: Hilary Tanner (Secretary to Mr Shilling)
To: Assistant to Managing Director, Brent Ankara
Re: Draft of itinerary and programme for President's visit

Number of pages, including this cover sheet: 1

1   Mr Shilling has to go to Paris on Friday and will fly Air France direct to Ankara from there (arr. 17.45)
2   Please note: Mrs Shilling will be accompanying her husband: change hotel booking accordingly.
3   Re: Sunday: They like museums; please make recommendations.
4   Re: Monday a.m. – Mr Shilling wants a breakfast meeting with the MD.
5   On Monday evening, Mr Shilling would like to invite the board out to dinner.
6   Tuesday morning: Mr Shilling wants to meet Sales and Marketing to discuss new product lines.

PS: Please note that Mr Shilling is a vegetarian

- Write a letter of **100–120 words** to Mr Shilling's secretary explaining the changes you have made to the original plan. Use the information above.
- You are advised to lay out your letter properly. The words in the address will not count in the 120 word limit.
- **Write on your Answer Sheet**.

LISTENING   Approximately 40 minutes (including 10 minutes transfer time)

PART ONE

Questions 1–12

- You will hear three recorded telephone messages.
- Write **one** or **two** words or a number in the numbered spaces on the forms below.
- After each message, rewind the tape and listen again.

Message One
(Questions 1–4)

- Look at the form below.
- You will hear a man ordering some items.

Product	Quantity	Product Title	Cost
Book	One	(1)	$24.95
(2)	Two	Building Teams	$200
Video	One	Competitive Strategies	(3) ....

Shipping and Handling within (4) ....: $18 per item $72

Name: John Hunt

Address: 601 Harmsworth Way, Boston, MA 02163, USA

Message Two
(Questions 5–8)

- Look at the form below.
- You will hear a woman asking for some information.

Date: 8.6.01
To: Oxford Management (5) ....
Attention: David (6) ....

Please send details of:
- The Oxford Management Programme
- (7) ....

Name: Caroline Lomas
Address: BC701, Core B, Hung Hom, Kowloon, Hong Kong

Tel: (852) 235 664485   e-mail: (8) ....

Message Three
(Questions 9–12)

● Look at the form below.
● You will hear a woman making a booking for an awards ceremony.

The Marketing Week Awards

celebrating 20 years of excellence, will take place on March 3, 1998 at the
(9) .... Hotel

☐ Please reserve a table for **(10)** .... @ £1,120.00
or
☐ Please reserve an individual place @ **(11)** ....

☐ Please send me a Dinner Booking Form

Name: Kari Mahmood   Job Title: **(12)** ....

Company: Apollo   Address: 23 Mercer Street,
                              Covent Garden, WC2H 9QB

Tel: 0171 674 2233   Fax: 0171 603 7884

PART TWO

Questions 13–22

Section One
(Questions 13–17)

● You will hear five people talking about their jobs.
● For each person, decide which type of job **A–H** they do.
● Write **one** letter **A–H** next to the number of the person.
● Do not use any letter more than once.
● At the end of question 17, rewind the tape and listen again.

13 ....

14 ....

15 ....

16 ....

17 ....

A	area manager
B	accountant
C	auctioneer
D	civil servant
E	lawyer
F	chief executive
G	dispatch rider
H	pilot

Section Two
(Questions 18–22)

- You will hear another five short pieces.
- For each piece, decide what task **A–H** the person is being asked to do.
- Write **one** letter **A–H** next to the number of the piece.
- At the end of question 22, rewind the tape and listen again.

18 ....

19 ....

20 ....

21 ....

22 ....

A	write a memo
B	produce a report
C	check some figures
D	offer a job
E	reply to a letter
F	make a telephone call
G	take some minutes
H	set up a database

PART THREE

Questions 23–30

- You will hear two people discussing Point of Purchasing (POP) projects.
- Choose the best phrase to answer or complete questions **23–30**.
- Mark **one** letter **A**, **B** or **C** for the phrase you choose.
- At the end of the talk, rewind the tape and listen again.

23 What do POP projects aim to do?

    A   encourage managers to plan their advertising

    B   increase sales of particular products

    C   increase the amount spent on advertising

24 Why has interest in POP been slow to develop?

    A   Most other forms of advertising are cheaper.

    B   The displays are difficult to set up.

    C   Managers need to make large initial investments.

25 What has made TV advertising less effective?

    A   The number of TV channels has increased.

    B   People are watching less TV these days.

    C   The quality of TV commercials is poor.

26 Samsung believes that POP will work for them because

    A   its products are of the best quality.
    B   customers can be persuaded to change their minds.
    C   other companies do not give value for money.

27 Some companies are investing in planning and research to

    A   encourage the use of POP.
    B   cut the costs of POP.
    C   assess the benefits of POP.

28 The Cheltenham and Gloucester Building Society improved their sales of pensions by

    A   offering well-designed leaflets and brochures.
    B   focusing advertising in specific physical areas.
    C   making better use of wall space for posters.

29 Why do large stores want to control POP campaigns?

    A   Stores may be unable to cope with demand.
    B   Stores do not approve of POP.
    C   Stores may sell less of their own products.

30 What is one of the problems facing POP agencies?

    A   There is a shortage of retail space.
    B   There are insufficient POP specialists.
    C   There is not enough interest in the medium.

**You now have 10 minutes to transfer your answers
to your Answer Sheet.**

SPEAKING   Approximately 12 minutes

Business guides
*For **two** candidates*

Candidate A

YOUR QUESTIONS

In this activity you will find out information about two guides to help you to run your own business. You will then discuss with your partner which one you would prefer to use. First find out more about the Business Start-Up Guide. Ask candidate B your questions.

1 Published by: ....

2 Content: ....

3 Contact: ....

Discussion:

Discuss with your partner which guide you would prefer to use. Consider what the guide is offering and any other details you think are important.

INFORMATION

Your partner will ask you questions about the One 2 One Business Guide. Use the information below to answer the questions.

One 2 One Business Guide
If you're in business, you'll find this book essential reading – and it's free!
◆ Are you running your own business and looking to expand?
◆ This book is full of useful contacts and helpful ideas.
◆ Contains hints on everything from management to marketing, staff training to taxation.
Produced by One 2 One in partnership with the Federation of Small Businesses.
For your free copy, call free on 0500 121 500
ONE 2 ONE
Our mobile phone service gets business talking

Business guides
*For **two** candidates*

Candidate B

YOUR QUESTIONS

In this activity you will find out information about two guides to help you to run your own business. You will then discuss with your partner which one you would prefer to use. First find out more about the One 2 One Business Guide. Ask candidate A your questions.

1 Aimed at? ....

2 Contains? ....

3 Produced by? ....

Discussion:

Discuss with your partner which guide you would prefer to use. Consider what the guide is offering and any other details you think are important.

INFORMATION

Your partner will ask you questions about the Business Start-Up Guide. Use the information below to answer the questions.

You've planned your new business.
Now write your business plan.

Page 18 shows you how

NatWest's comprehensive Business Start-Up Guide covers many of the things you should remember before going it alone.
Everything from writing a business plan to legal considerations.
For your FREE copy why not contact your local business adviser? With at least one in each of our high street branches you've over 4,000 to choose from or
Call 0800 777 888

NatWest
More than just a bank

KEY

Test 1 Reading

Each correct answer is worth 1 mark (total 45).

Part One

1 D   2 A   3 D   4 C   5 C   6 A
7 B

Part Two

8 D   9 I   10 H   11 B   12 E

Part Three

13 A   14 G   15 E   16 F
17 A   18 D   19 B   20 F

Part Four

21 D   22 A   23 B   24 A   25 C
26 C   27 D   28 A   29 C   30 D
31 A   32 B   33 B   34 D   35 C

Part Five

36 for   37 so   38 ✔   39 they   40 very
41 your   should be   you're/you are
42 can pushing   should be   can push
43 This shelf also have   should be   This shelf
also has
44 comfortable   should be   comfort
45 the chair what is   should be   the chair that/
which is

Test 1 Writing

Anything in ( ) brackets is optional. Alternative
answers are separated by / /. Open-ended
completions are in [ ] brackets.

Part One (10 marks)

Question 46 Specimen answer

To   Head of Department
From   Char Shui
Re   Diskflow pump
Where
I (have) read about the Diskflow pump in [name
of source, e.g. the Pump Times].
Why a good investment
It needs very little maintenance and could save the
company a lot of money.

Offer to find out more
If you want/are interested, I could [source of
further info, e.g. write to Diskflow Company for
more information].

[38 words, excluding underlined headings]

Part Two (15 marks)

Question 47 Specimen answer

To   Conference Organiser
From   Secretary, CADE Hazards, Birmingham
Date   [date before 30.05, e.g. 28 May 1999]
Re   Arrangements for CADE Hazards
            one-day conference

Change the date of the conference to 4 June and
use the Natt Conference Centre.
Tell Natt that we expect 38 participants, including
myself and the Group Chairman.
Book five single rooms at the local hotel for the
night of 4 June.
Contact Jerry in Accounts to arrange advance
payment. Note that guests will be responsible for
extras, e.g. phone calls, minibar.
Book two cars with Sid's Cabs for transfer of five
participants from railway station to Conference
Centre. They will pay the cab driver.
I confirm that there will be a tenth anniversary
dinner at the Centre on the evening of 4 June.
Make a booking for 38 people.

[111 words, excluding headings]

Test 1 Listening

You are given 1 mark for each correct answer. The
total number of marks available for the listening
paper is 30.

Part One (Questions 1–12)

(1 mark for each correct answer)

1	Construction	7	$160
2	4.30 p.m./in the afternoon	8	1456 7682
3	statement	9	laptop
4	items/things/large sums	10	$400
5	18 June/18/6	11	delivery
6	non-smoking	12	6758241

Part Two (Questions 13–22)

13	C	18	G
14	F	19	D
15	D	20	C
16	G	21	A
17	E	22	E

Part Three (Questions 23–30)

23	C	27	A
24	B	28	B
25	A	29	C
26	B	30	B

Tapescript

Listening Test One

Practice Tests for the Cambridge Business English Certificate Level 2. Listening Test 1.

PART 1

Part One. Questions 1 to 12.

You will hear three recorded telephone messages. Write one or two words or a number in the numbered spaces on the forms below.
After each message, rewind the tape and listen again.

Message 1

Message One. Questions 1 to 4.

Look at the form below. You will hear a man leaving a message for his bank.

You have 15 seconds to read through the form.

[pause]

Now listen and fill in the spaces.

Man: This is Lewis Bradfield speaking, from Collings Construction Company, and I'm phoning today, that's Tuesday, February 14th and it's 4.30 in the afternoon.
Actually I thought there'd be someone there. Still, never mind. What I'm phoning about is that I got this statement from you today. It's my business account you know. And, well, there are a few items on it that I don't understand. I mean there are several items which have been debited to the account which I simply don't recognise. It's very worrying. So please, could you get back to me as soon as possible. Well, today if you can. Er, thanks.

[pause]

Now rewind the tape and listen again.

[pause]

Message 2

Message Two. Questions 5 to 8.

Look at the form below. You will hear a hotel manager leaving a message for Mr Lacey.

You have 15 seconds to read through the form.

[pause]

Now listen and fill in the spaces.

Woman: Good morning. This is the Mandarin Court Hotel in Shanghai. I would like to leave a message for Mr Lacey. It's 8th June here in Shanghai. My name is Madame Li.
I would just like to confirm that we are expecting Mr Lacey on 12th June and that his reservation with us will be until 18th June. We have given him a non-smoking room on the 14th floor as you requested.
The room rate is normally $185 a night but we would like to offer Mr Lacey the room for only $160.
Please let us know if there is anything else Mr Lacey requires. Our fax and phone number is 86 21 1456 7682. Thank you for making this reservation with us.

[pause]

Now rewind the tape and listen again.

[pause]

Message 3

Message Three. Questions 9 to 12.

Look at the form below. You will hear a man from a computer rental company leaving a message.

You have 15 seconds to read through the form.

[pause]

Now listen and fill in the spaces.

Man: It's Computer Rental Services, Jim Darma speaking. I'd like to leave a message for Dr Adams. Could you let him know that we do have a laptop p.c. available for rent. The cost is $400 per month and insurance is extra. We'd need to know whether he will be taking it out of the country or not. Could he let us know what day he wants it delivered? I'd also be grateful if he could get back to me, that's Jim Darma, today please on 675 8241. That's a local number. Thanks. Goodbye.

[pause]

Now rewind the tape and listen again.

[pause]

That is the end of Part One. You now have 20 seconds to check your answers.

[pause]

PART 2

Part Two. Questions 13 to 22.

Section 1

Section One. Questions 13 to 17.

You will hear five people talking about different items.
For each piece, decide which item A to H the speaker is talking about.
Write one letter A to H next to the number of the piece.
Do not use any letter more than once.

At the end of question 17, rewind the tape and listen again.

You have 15 seconds to read the list of items A to H.

[pause]

Now listen and decide what each speaker is talking about.

[pause]

Question 13 *Thirteen*

Woman: Joe, I've got Mr Brand on the line and he says he hasn't got the cheque for his trip yet. Apparently he had to pay the hotel in cash and it was quite a lot of money. Do you know if his form has been processed yet?

[pause]

Question 14 *Fourteen*

Man: We are going to start the campaign by putting full-page ads in all the major newspapers over a period of a month. They'll be in weekly, probably on a Monday, and after that we are planning to focus on TV and Radio.

[pause]

Question 15 *Fifteen*

Woman: Mr Carpenter has decided to postpone it until after the next consignment has gone out. I shall fax everyone who was due to come and give them some alternative dates.

[pause]

Question 16 *Sixteen*

Man: I shall be coming round to each of you to discuss how you think things have gone so far. I'm going to need as much detail as possible because I want the documentation to be a realistic record of events.

[pause]

Question 17 *Seventeen*

Woman: It's a very sophisticated model. You can programme it to send stuff at any time and then if there's a problem a message appears on this little screen here. It even suggests what you can do about it to put it right!

[pause]

Now rewind the tape and listen again.

[pause]

Section 2

Section Two. Questions 18 to 22.

You will hear another five short pieces.
For each piece, decide who the speaker is.
Write one letter A to H next to the number of the piece.
Do not use any letter more than once.

At the end of question 22, rewind the tape and listen again.

You have 15 seconds to read the list of jobs A to H.

[pause]

Now listen and decide who is speaking.

[pause]

Question 18 *Eighteen*

Man: Could you tell me where the talk on International Banking is going to take place? It says in the programme that it's in Room 121 but I've just been up there and it's empty. I hope it hasn't been cancelled.

[pause]

Question 19 *Nineteen*

Woman: Here is your key Mrs Perez. You are on the 14th floor, overlooking the river. Would you like me to reserve you a table in our restaurant this evening?

[pause]

Question 20 *Twenty*

Man: Unfortunately, sir, we can't let anybody into the building without an identification pass. If you could just wait a moment, I'll call Mr Blair's office and see if his secretary can help.

[pause]

Question 21 *Twenty-one*

Man: Oh dear, I've just heard we are going to be without telephones this afternoon while they are installing the new system. I'd better let the manager know immediately as she said she was going to ring me from the airport with that report she wants sent out.

[pause]

Question 22 *Twenty-two*

Woman: I'm afraid I won't be able to make that meeting today, Jane. I've got appointments all morning and then head office wants me to discuss interest rates at the board meeting. I need time to get the figures together.

[pause]

Now rewind the tape and listen again.

[pause]

That is the end of Part Two.

[pause]

PART 3

Part Three. Questions 23 to 30.

You will hear a woman giving advice on how to give a good presentation.
Choose the best phrase to answer or complete questions 23 to 30.
Mark one letter A, B or C for the sentence you choose.

At the end of the talk, rewind the tape and listen again.

You have 45 seconds to read through the questions.

[pause]

Now listen and mark A, B or C.

[pause]

Woman: When you're making a presentation, your posture can affect the quality of your voice. The way you stand, you know, the position of your head, neck and shoulders and feet and so on is important. Check that your feet are parallel and apart and your weight is slightly forward on your feet. Make sure that your knees are relaxed, as if you are tense your back will suffer. Pay special attention to your head. Look straight ahead and don't push your neck out or drop it on to your chest. I had a man come to see me once as he was constantly losing his voice. It was all due to his habit of sticking his neck forward which was putting pressure on his throat. He sounded quite squeaky when he spoke. What he should have been doing was keeping his ears in line with his shoulders. Your head should feel as though it's floating on top of your body! So watch that.

Now most of us feel quite nervous before we speak in public. You'll feel better if you spend some time dealing with the tension. It's a good idea to try and think about what it is that's making you feel this way. That way you can have some control over it. Next, try and locate the area of tension in your body. Often it's your neck or your shoulders. Then concentrate on massaging these parts and consciously trying to relax them. Believe me, it works!

Let's think about what you say, now. To maximise your performance make sure you are well-prepared. Look over your notes, practise what you want to say, preferably out loud, and then, perhaps most important of all, try to feel you really want to share your subject with your audience. If you feel and share your enthusiasm with them, you're more than half-way there.

Remember that how people feel about you and what you are saying to them will depend on your body language. There are three main behaviour types: Passive, Aggressive and Assertive. You can use any of these types, although I think the assertive posture is one that suits most occasions best.

The passive body type has a withdrawn posture. You may fidget a bit with your hands and hair.

In fact I remember a well-known politician who whenever he was speaking would constantly massage the top of his head. So beware of those funny little mannerisms. They can become intensely irritating to an audience.

If your posture is aggressive, however, you tend to be quite rigid. You could be constantly swinging your leg or crossing your arms and clenching your fists and the audience will feel uncomfortable. Your voice will often sound harsh or sharp and your audience may then feel quite aggressive towards you and that's something you don't want if your aim is to get them to see your point of view.

That brings me to the assertive posture. Now you're standing straight, feeling comfortable and calm with your arms hanging loosely at your sides. In this position there is minimal tension and your voice is full, clear and varied. You're a delight to listen to.

Finally, a few do's and don'ts when it comes to looking after your voice, especially before giving a speech or whatever. It's a bit obvious but avoid smoky areas, and alcohol, too. Drink plenty of fluids, especially things like fruit juice or even coffee or tea and keep your throat moist while you're speaking. Also, interestingly enough, stop eating too many dairy products when you have a cold. It can make you sound worse – and also don't forget to use your lips and tongue carefully to make the words stand out clearly.

And just a final reminder. We can't always control the room we are speaking in. So, if a plane goes over, don't shout. Wait till it's gone. Don't battle with things you can't do anything about. If your throat feels uncomfortable, try not to cough violently or clear your throat. Just swallow instead. It doesn't always work but it's much better for your voice.

That's it, ladies and gentlemen. We shall be going on to do some exercises to help you relax now. If you can gather round ...

[pause]

Now rewind the tape and listen again.

[pause]

That is the end of Part Three. You now have ten minutes to transfer your answers to your Answer Sheet. [**Teachers:** Time 9 minutes starting now.]

[pause]

You have one more minute.

[pause]

That is the end of the test.

Test 2   Reading

Each correct answer is worth 1 mark (total 45).

Part One

1 B	2 D	3 C	4 A	5 B	6 A
7 D					

Part Two

8 G	9 D	10 F	11 A	12 H

Part Three

13 C	14 E	15 G	16 A
17 E	18 G	19 C	20 A

Part Four

21 B	22 C	23 A	24 D	25 D
26 B	27 A	28 C	29 C	30 A
31 B	32 B	33 D	34 C	35 D

Part 5

36 been	37 ✔	38 with	39 the	40 which

41 likelihood   should be   likely
42 damaged   should be   damage
43 no   should be   any
44 other's   should be   other
45 easy   should be   easily

Test 2   Writing

Anything in ( ) brackets is optional. Alternative answers are separated by / /. Open-ended completions are in [ ] brackets.

Part One (10 marks)

Question 46 Specimen answer

To   All staff
From   Manager
Re   Use of telephones
Costs
Recent telephone bills have been very high.
Length of calls
I must ask all of you not to make long phone calls/ to keep your calls as short as possible.
Personal use of phones

Please note that office telephones are not to be used to make personal calls.
<u>Conclusion</u> (optional)
Thank you for your cooperation.

[38 words, excluding underlined headings]

Part Two (15 marks)

Question 47 Specimen answer

[your address]

James Carter, Sales
Better Business Systems
BBS House
Dawley Business Park
Telford TF34 3JJ

[date]

Dear Mr Carter

Re: **Order for office furniture**

Thank you for your confirmation of our order. We want to make a few changes to our order. First, we confirm that the filing cabinets should be grey, but we want the desks and the bookcases in beige. Secondly, we wish to change the order for typists' chairs to chairs without arms. Thirdly, please note that we wish to order 4, not 3, filing cabinets. The delivery date is satisfactory, but can you confirm that you will be able to make the deliver in the morning?

Our MD cannot manage the date you suggest for the site meeting. Could your secretary phone his secretary, [name], to arrange another time?

Thank you for your attention to these changes.
Yours sincerely
[your name]
Purchasing Officer

[119 words, excluding headings]

Test 2   Listening

You are given 1 mark for each correct answer. The total number of marks available for the listening paper is 30.

Part One (Questions 1–12)

(1 mark for each correct answer)
1 (experienced) receptionist
2 communication/(good) communicator
3 word processing
4 July
5 Sales
6 Saturday
7 executive
8 catering staff
9 Mr Brown
10 lunch
11 factory
12 accountant

Part Two (Questions 13–22)

13	A	18	D
14	E	19	B
15	C	20	C
16	B	21	G
17	H	22	E

Part Three (Questions 23–30)

23	A	27	A
24	C	28	A
25	B	29	C
26	B	30	A

Tapescript

Listening Test Two

Practice Tests for the Cambridge Business English Certificate Level 2. Listening Test 2.

PART 1

Part One. Questions 1 to 12.

You will hear three telephone conversations. Write one or two words in the numbered spaces on the forms below.
After each conversation, rewind the tape and listen again.

Conversation 1

Conversation 1. Questions 1 to 4.

Look at the form below. You will hear a woman talking to an employment agency.

You have 15 seconds to read through the form.

[pause]

Now listen and fill in the spaces.

Woman: Hello. Is that the Personplan employment agency?
Man: Yes, it is. How can I help you?
Woman: I'm Janet Cross from Universal Lift Incorporated. We need an experienced receptionist who's a good communicator. The person must be able to use a word processor as well.
Man: I think we can do something about that. You'll be wanting them to start ...?
Woman: Um, well, July would suit us best. Our receptionist is planning to leave in August and we want her to show the new person the ropes.

Man: Very sensible. If you'll just give me a few more details, I'll see what we can do for you . . .

[pause]

Now rewind the tape and listen again.

[pause]

Conversation 2

Conversation Two. Questions 5 to 8.

Look at the form below. You will hear a man talking to a catering services department.

You have 15 seconds to read through the form.

[pause]

Now listen and fill in the spaces.

Man: Good morning, is that Victoria in Catering? It's Moss from Sales Division here.

Woman: No, Mr Moss, I'm afraid she's not here at the moment. Can I take a message?

Man: Well, I want to order a dinner for the reps on Saturday. Now, there's going to be eight of them and seven from here so we are looking at 15. With that sort of size it's going to have to be the executive dining room as the board room isn't big enough, don't you think? And then I want at least three catering staff on duty. That should do it. Now food –

Woman: I think I ought to check that through with Victoria and get back to you with the menus, really –

Man: Yes, yes. You're probably right . . .

[pause]

Now rewind the tape and listen again.

[pause]

Conversation 3

Conversation Three. Questions 9 to 12.

Look at the diary below. You will hear two people discussing appointments.

You have 15 seconds to read through the form.

[pause]

Now listen and fill in the spaces.

Woman: What's next week looking like, Ben? I want to find time to go over that report with you.

Man: I'm just looking at the diary and as far as I can see you're not free until Wednesday

morning. You've got that meeting with Mr Brown on Monday at 9.30 and then there's Lee Van Canh for lunch and that's bound to go on most of the afternoon. Tuesday's out as you're at the factory all day. So it's going to have to be Wednesday morning. And don't forget that you have an appointment at quarter past two with the accountant so we'll have to cut it short before lunch. Looks like another busy week!

[pause]

Now rewind the tape and listen again.

[pause]

That is the end of Part One. You now have 20 seconds to check your answers.

[pause]

PART 2

Part Two. Questions 13 to 22.

Section 1

Section One. Questions 13 to 17.

You will hear five short advertisements. For each piece, decide which topic A to H the speaker is talking about. Write one letter A to H next to the number of the piece. Do not use any letter more than once

At the end of question 17, rewind the tape and listen again.

You have 15 seconds to read the list of topics A to H.

[pause]

Now listen and decide what each speaker is talking about.

[pause]

Question 13 *Thirteen*

Man: We have over 40 years' experience of supplying leading companies throughout the world. We produce a top-class product to enhance the image of your company without costing the earth. We are very proud of our reputation for personal service and reliability and your order will receive immediate attention and be delivered on time, every time. It's the only way we know.

[pause]

Question 14 *Fourteen*

Woman: Are you looking for the perfect person for your annual corporate event? We can provide you with whatever suits the occasion from knowledgeable expert to glamorous celebrity. As you know, it's what they say *and* how they say it. We can advise on and deliver unforgettable presentations or spell-binding story-telling. Call us.

[pause]

Question 15 *Fifteen*

Woman: The Foxley Halls complex boasts a reputation for service and excellence second to none. We offer all the facilities you will need and are within easy access to all major routes. We have ample car parking, superb catering and all this in the traditional surroundings of a historical setting and relaxing countryside. Impress your clients, stimulate your trainees or simply provide a beautiful background to display your products.

[pause]

Question 16 *Sixteen*

Woman: Suitable for new or soon to be promoted management, the emphasis in this programme is on people management. We'll give you clear guidelines, explicit case studies, exercises, presentations and evening syndicate work. The focus is on reality and what can and cannot be done in the actual business environment.

[pause]

Question 17 *Seventeen*

Man: Whether in our personal or business lives, we are all at risk of having our privacy invaded. We can offer a range of products designed to reduce the possibility of unwanted intrusion. Visit our new showroom for the latest specialist innovations including listening devices, communications equipment, personal protection, video cameras and much more.

[pause]

Now rewind the tape and listen again.

[pause]

Section 2

Section Two. Questions 18 to 22.

You will hear five speakers talking about different departments of an organisation.
For each piece, decide which department A to H the speaker is talking about.
Write one letter A to H next to the number of the piece.
Do not use any letter more than once.

At the end of question 22, rewind the tape and listen again.

You have 15 seconds to read the list of departments A to H.

[pause]

Now listen and decide which department of the organisation each speaker is talking about.

[pause]

Question 18 *Eighteen*

Man: There's just the two of us in here and it can get very tense, especially as we get towards the end of the month. It's absolutely vital that everything is completed to schedule otherwise the staff won't get paid on time. There's no bigger disaster than that, is there?

[pause]

Question 19 *Nineteen*

Woman: We've had a big problem lately with screen savers. Lots of staff like to load these and several times the whole system has gone down or else there's been a virus. Well, they've been banned completely now, and we just have to hope that the staff do as they are told. Yes, we have to monitor things very carefully from here.

[pause]

Question 20 *Twenty*

Man: We work in a large open-plan setting which can be tricky at times with the sort of work we do. There are small meeting rooms where we can go to discuss things confidentially or where members of staff can talk to us in private. Of course, with the sort of information we keep, individual staff records and interview reports and so on, we have to be discreet at all times.

[pause]

Question 21 *Twenty-one*

Woman: It can get extremely noisy down here.

89

The staff are supposed to wear ear protectors at all times but that's impossible if you need to talk to someone. The other thing we have to contend with is dirt and dust. It's OK when we're not too busy but when there's a rush on there isn't time to clear up.

[pause]

Question 22 *Twenty-two*

Man: We offer a very personalised service to the different divisions. Some of the staff are dedicated to groups of individuals within these divisions. That way we get to know what sort of service they are looking for and how much help they need from us over conference organisation or brochures or whatever. What we do insist on, whether it's leaflets or posters or local information, is quality.

[pause]

Now rewind the tape and listen again.

[pause]

That is the end of Part Two.

[pause]

PART 3

Part Three. Questions 23 to 30.

You will hear an interview with Carol Vogel, the President of Telekom. She is talking about their current situation and future prospects.
Choose the best phrase to answer or complete questions 23 to 30.
Mark one letter A, B or C for the answer you choose.

At the end of the interview, rewind the tape and listen again.

You have 45 seconds to read through the questions.

[pause]

Now listen and mark A, B or C.

[pause]

Interviewer: Welcome to the studio, Ms Vogel. As President of Telekom you have been in a difficult position over the last few months of financial uncertainty in the region. How tough has it been?
Carol Vogel: I want to be positive and see the current situation as a challenge. The capital requirements of Telekom's infrastructure are enormous. The recent currency turmoil is bound to slow down investment in the short term, but it is unlikely to reduce its total volume in the long term.
Interviewer: But isn't it the case that some of your projects have been delayed?
Carol: Yes, but not cancelled. Our advisers are telling us that a temporary reduction in the number of new projects is not serious. We still have many ongoing contracts with foreign operators which do not come up for renewal until 2010.
Interviewer: But it appears that you have several major challenges in your effort to upgrade the telecommunications network in this country.
Carol: Yes, that is true. I see three major challenges. The first is the nature of our country. We are a country of several thousand islands: this presents a unique problem for the existing technology to deal with. Secondly, there is the question of affordability. We have a relatively low GDP per capita, $1,132 by the end of 1998. And finally funds – it costs between $1,000 and $1,200 to put in a line.
Interviewer: Yes, I believe that there are fewer than three lines per 100 people.
Carol: There are plans which will go ahead to install 6 million lines by the end of the year which will improve this figure to around five lines for every 100 people. In the West the average is about 60 lines per 100 people.
Interviewer: So there is a long way to go. Is the government playing its part?
Carol: The government has been very supportive. By allowing the industry to become privatised there has been much progress. It acted very sensibly and compared to other countries in the region it has worked very well. Our relationship with the government and other telecommunications' operators is good.
Interviewer: You are referring to the huge international group investors?
Carol: Yes. In 1995, five international groups committed themselves to the development of the telecommunications infrastructure in five regions of the country. Each group agreed to install a target number of lines and operate them for 15 years and then return them to Telekom.
Interviewer: And it looks as if the private sector development is also well-established in the mobile communications sector?

Carol: The number of subscribers has jumped to 562,500 from 25,000 two years ago. There are three competing suppliers. Each of these three operations is a joint venture with ourselves. This is an area which is seeing major growth throughout Asia. We are glad to be part of it.

Interviewer: So in your view there is not too much to worry about?

Carol: There are plenty of issues that need to be resolved but I am sure that the good times will return and this can only mean that Telekom will prosper in the long run.

[pause]

Now rewind the tape and listen again.

[pause]

That is the end of Part Three. You now have ten minutes to transfer your answers to your Answer Sheet. [**Teachers:** Time 9 minutes starting now.]

[pause]

You have one more minute.

[pause]

That is the end of the test.

Test 3 Reading

Each correct answer is worth 1 mark (total 45).

Part One

1 C   2 B   3 C   4 A   5 B   6 D
7 A

Part Two

8 D   9 F   10 A   11 I   12 B

Part Three

13 C   14 G   15 A   16 E
17 G   18 B   19 E   20 A

Part Four

21 B   22 D   23 D   24 A   25 D
26 A   27 C   28 B   29 D   30 B
31 C   32 C   33 B   34 C   35 A

Part Five

36 of   37 ✔   38 it   39 as   40 one
41 businesses   should be   business
42 exceed   should be   excess
43 incur   should be   incurs

44 entry   should be   enter
45 who's   should be   whose

Test 3 Writing

Anything in ( ) brackets is optional. Alternative answers are separated by / /. Open-ended completions are in [ ] brackets.

Part One (10 marks)

Question 46 Specimen answer

To   The Managing Director (or similar title)
From   Chief Accountant
Re   Smart Finance training course
Request
I should like to attend this course about a new financial management program.
Course details
The course is on [23 September] and costs [US$500].
Usefulness
I think that attending this course will help me to do my job better in future.

[38 words, excluding underlined headings]

Part Two (15 marks)

Question 47 Specimen answer

Mrs Morton
Flash Move International
Head Office
Carter House
Lade Way
Cambridge CB9 1EE

[date]

Dear Mrs Morton

Re: Office move

Thank you for your reply of [date]. We accept your removal costs, but need to change the date from mid-May to October. Please confirm that you can do this. Could you also confirm that the cost of packing includes any fragile equipment we have? We need to know, too, exactly what your insurance covers. Please note that we have decided not to store any furniture with you after all. Finally, the date you suggest for your visit is not convenient. Could we change it to [alternative date]? Please phone me if this is not suitable. We look forward to hearing from you at your earliest convenience.
Yours sincerely

[111 words, excluding headings]

Test 3   Listening

You are given 1 mark for each correct answer. The total number of marks available for the listening paper is 30.

Part One (Questions 1–12)

(1 mark for each correct answer)

1	Dr Rae	7	overdrawn
2	Finance	8	(£)200
3	Friday / 11.30	9	Hong Kong
4	taxi	10	short/difficult/tight
5	account/number	11	5 hour
6	cheque	12	first class

Part Two (Questions 13–22)

13	B	18	C
14	D	19	D
15	F	20	G
16	C	21	B
17	H	22	F

Part Three (Questions 23–30)

23	A	27	A
24	B	28	C
25	C	29	C
26	C	30	A

Tapescript

Listening Test Three

Practice Tests for the Cambridge Business English Certificate Level 2. Listening Test 3.

PART 1

Part One. Questions 1 to 12.

You will hear three telephone conversations. Write one or two words or a number in the numbered spaces on the forms below.
At the end of each conversation, rewind the tape and listen again.

Conversation 1

Conversation One. Questions 1 to 4.

Look at the form below. A woman is leaving instructions for her assistant.

You have 15 seconds to read through the form.

[pause]

Now listen and fill in the spaces.

Woman: I've got to dash off and catch a train, Joe. Could you make sure that when Mr Rae calls – you know, the new IT consultant – that I want him to start with networking the computers in the marketing division. He may want to start with the finance group but he can do that afterwards. I'm anxious we get marketing started.

Man: Sure. I think it's *Dr* Rae – R-A-E, isn't it?

Woman: Yes, you're right. Also I want to see James about the shareholders' meeting. Look in my diary . . . I think I'm free on Friday at 10 a.m.?

Man: No, you've got a meeting but you should be through by 11. I'll pencil him in for 11.30.

Woman: Fine. Now I must go. If you want you can get me at Regent House this afternoon.

Man: Yes. Do you want a taxi to pick you up this evening?

Woman: Yes, please. I'll let you know what time . . . I'm off!

Man: Bye. I'll call you.

Woman: Thanks, Joe. Bye.

Man: Bye, Rachel. Have a good day.

[pause]

Now rewind the tape and listen again.

[pause]

Conversation 2

Conversation Two. Questions 5 to 8.

Look at the form below. You will hear a man complaining to his bank.

You have 15 seconds to read through the form.

[pause]

Now listen and fill in the spaces.

Man 1: There's several things I'm not happy about, Mr Simms. First of all –

Man 2: Do you mind if I take some notes? Could you give me your name and account number?

Man 1: I'm Frank Bailey and the number's 5220 4768. The first thing is that I asked for that cheque for £2,000 to be paid into my current account, and it wasn't. It went into my deposit account. So then I was overdrawn and next thing is I get a letter from you telling me you're charging me for this.

Man 2: Oh dear, perhaps there was some confusion –

Man 1: And it gets worse. I now find that someone has taken £200 out of my account.

Man 2: That's very serious –

Man 1: And just to cap it all I find I can't use my cash-point card. The machine spits it out!

Man 2: It sounds as though we have some serious problems here. If you could just give me a moment . . .

[pause]

Now rewind the tape and listen again.

[pause]

Conversation 3

Conversation Three. Questions 9 to 12.

Look at the form below. You will hear a woman talking about flight arrangements.

You have 15 seconds to read through the form.

[pause]

Now listen and fill in the spaces.

Woman 1: I've got some details about possible flights for Ms Burton.

Woman 2: Oh good, she's been waiting for those.

Woman 1: There's a choice of flights out but some of the transfer times are not great. There's a BA flight at 21.30 arriving Hong Kong at 17.40 where she can pick up the 19.10 KLM flight to Manila.

Woman 2: Sounds a bit tight. That's only one and a half hours to transfer.

Woman 1: The alternative is to fly to Amsterdam and get a direct flight from there. The disadvantage with that one is that there are no seats at the moment . . . she'd have to be wait-listed. Also it's a five-hour wait at Amsterdam. Coming back's no problem. There's a Cathay flight all the way and as they have no business seats they've offered her a first class seat at no extra cost!

Woman 2: Great! She'll enjoy that.

[pause]

Now rewind the tape and listen again.

[pause]

That is the end of Part One. You now have 20 seconds to check your answers.

[pause]

PART 2

Part Two. Questions 13 to 22.

Section 1

Section One. Questions 13 to 17.

You will hear five people talking in different places.
For each piece, choose the location A to H where the person is speaking.
Write one letter A to H next to the number of the piece.
Do not use any letter more than once.

After question 17, rewind the tape and listen again.

You have 15 seconds to read the list of locations A to H.

[pause]

Now listen and decide where each speaker is speaking.

[pause]

Question 13 *Thirteen*

Woman: Ah yes, you are Ian Woodward? You've brought some clothes and things with you, I see. Good. You'll probably be in for a few days at least. I'm afraid there's going to be a bit of a wait as your bed's not ready yet. The last patient only left an hour ago.

[pause]

Question 14 *Fourteen*

Man: You'll never guess what's happened! They've lost my luggage. It was checked through all the way so I haven't seen it since I left London. I'll have to go and fill in some forms over there, I suppose.

[pause]

Question 15 *Fifteen*

Woman: I don't think we've got any left, sir, but I'll check in the store at the back if you'll wait a minute. Yes, there's been quite a run on them this week. It must be all this hot weather we're having.

[pause]

Question 16 *Sixteen*

Man: I don't know how you can concentrate with

all this noise, but I suppose you get used to it. Could you tell me how to get to the foreman's office, please?

[pause]

Question 17 *Seventeen*

Woman: Can you see a space anywhere? This is the trouble with coming into work late. Well, I'm just going to have to use the director's place. I think she's away, anyway.

[pause]

Now rewind the tape and listen again.

[pause]

Section 2

Section Two. Questions 18 to 22.

You will hear five people talking on the phone. For each piece, decide the reason A to H for the telephone call.
Write one letter A to H next to the number of the piece.
Do not use any letter more than once.

At the end of question 22, rewind the tape and listen again.

You have 15 seconds to read the list of reasons A to H.

[pause]

Now listen and decide why each speaker is calling.

[pause]

Question 18 *Eighteen*

Man: I just wanted to say well done for getting that contract. You did a great job and we know it wasn't easy. What would you say to a celebratory meal? I know a very good restaurant near here. I'm sure we could get a table for lunch if you're free.

[pause]

Question 19 *Nineteen*

Man: Are you going to Head office on Monday? If you are, do you want to go with me? I could pick you up about 8 and we'd be there by 10 if there wasn't too much traffic. What do you say?

[pause]

Question 20 *Twenty*

Woman: Is that Rosie? Hi there. Do you think you

could do me a favour? I'm supposed to be seeing the boss this afternoon but something's come up. Actually, I'm going out to dinner. Could you make some sort of sensible excuse and say I'll catch up with him on Monday? Thanks a lot.

[pause]

Question 21 *Twenty-one*

Woman: I'm coming in for a meeting with Mr Savage today at 10 and I just wanted to be sure that I know how to reach you. Are you in that large building at the corner of Station Road? It's called Cintra House, or something?

[pause]

Question 22 *Twenty-two*

Man: Well, if you haven't any left in that colour, I don't think I'll bother. What about the trousers on page 14? Have you got those in a medium size? I'll have two pairs of them in grey, please. Do you charge for postage and packing?

[pause]

Now rewind the tape and listen again.

[pause]

That is the end of Part Two.

[pause]

PART 3

Part Three. Questions 23 to 30.

You will hear Paul talk about how he set up his own business to advise companies about their information technology needs.
Choose the best phrase to answer or complete questions 23 to 30.
Mark one letter A, B or C for the answer you choose.

At the end of the talk, rewind the tape and listen again.

You have 45 seconds to read through the questions.

[pause]

Now listen and mark A, B or C.

[pause]

Man: Many businesses get in a mess when they are setting up because they buy in a whole load of computers and fancy gadgets, get on the Internet and then start to panic. I believe that the biggest threat to businesses today is not having a clue about information technology and what it can and can't do for them. The company I have set up has one aim which is to solve your 'hidden' problem. We cover everything from complex cable infrastructures to setting up work-stations and servers.

Sometimes they see how much we charge and step back saying they are too small to need this sort of help. Yes, we are expensive and no, we haven't been in this business for hundreds of years. Nobody has and that's the point. This is a relatively new area and we can't show them a list of prestigious clients who have used our services, at least, not yet.

Of course lots of companies will offer you advice and expensive consultancy but they don't stay around to see you through the difficult bit. Once we have agreed terms my team go in, look at the technology requirements, advise them on it and then, crucially, go ahead and implement those needs. We're a bit like a management consultancy, but we do the whole thing – we give them a total business solution. We don't have a stock of products we sell. What we give the customer is more of a business expertise package.

I learnt the hard way. My first attempt to set up my own computer research company was a spectacular disaster, after I fell out with my business partner. Unfortunately I gave him 50% of the shares. We had a major argument about how much to invest to expand the business and then despite the success of the company it all fell apart. The saddest thing was having to sack a very enthusiastic bunch of staff.

So this time I think I've learnt my lesson. I started the company in my garage. In three years it has built up to 20 staff and a £4 million turnover with projected profits this year of £300,000. There's only me taking the risks but my staff are behind me and we've moved out of the garage! I think it's clear to everybody who works for me that I am not just letting the company potter along. We are dynamic and look ahead. I think that inspires people who join us and also they know that I discuss things with them even though I make the decisions.

The most satisfying thing right now is that I have a company with a clear mission. It's relatively successful and fast-growing. Although I was a skilled finance person, I've had to develop a lot of technical and sales skills so I'm a bit of an all-rounder now. I have to be honest and say that in five years' time I don't want to be doing this. It's not that I want to give up work and live in the country, but my plan is to move on and do something different. Not another business but another lifestyle. I could do that. This should be worth up to £25 million by then.

[pause]

Now rewind the tape and listen again.

[pause]

That is the end of Part Three. You now have ten minutes to transfer your answers to your Answer Sheet. [**Teachers:** Time 9 minutes starting now.]

[pause]

You have one more minute.

[pause]

That is the end of the test.

Test 4   Reading

Each correct answer is worth 1 mark (total 45).

Part One

1 D   2 A   3 C   4 B   5 C   6 D
7 B

Part Two

8 D   9 A   10 I   11 C   12 F

Part Three

13 C   14 B   15 F   16 D
17 B   18 F   19 D   20 G

Part Four

21 B   22 C   23 D   24 A   25 D
26 B   27 C   28 A   29 B   30 D
31 D   32 D   33 C   34 B   35 A

Part Five

36 off   37 as   38 ✔   39 any   40 its
41 print   should be   printed
42 during   should be   while
43 necessity   should be   necessary
44 for   should be   in
45 attaching   should be   attached

Test 4   Writing

Anything in ( ) brackets is optional. Alternative answers are separated by / /. Open-ended completions are in [ ] brackets.

Part One (10 marks)

Question 46 Specimen answer

To   Secretary to Señor Viladomat
From   [your company]
Re   Your visit to [name of company]
<u>Travel</u>
Our driver will meet him at the airport [+ time] and take him to the [hotel name],
<u>Accommodation</u>
where we have booked a single room for him.
<u>Meeting</u>
The meeting is at our head office on [day] starting at [time].

[38 words, excluding underlined headings]

Part Two (15 marks)

Question 47 Specimen answer

                                            [your address]
Hilary Tanner
Brent Pharmaceuticals
Poole House
Bridge Street SE23 5RT
                                            [date]
Dear Hilary

Re: Mr Shilling's visit to Ankara

Thank you for your fax. We have made the changes you requested. We note that Mr Shilling is flying direct to Ankara with Air France, and we have arranged for our driver to meet the flight. We have changed the hotel booking to a double room. On Sunday, we think they should visit the [name of museum] because it contains many interesting things. For Monday evening, we have booked a table for [number of people] at the [name of restaurant], which also does vegetarian dishes. We confirm that the Sales and Marketing staff will be available on Tuesday morning for a meeting with Mr Shilling.

Yours sincerely
[your name]
[title]

[111 words, excluding headings]

Test 4   Listening

You are given 1 mark for each correct answer. The total number of marks available for the listening paper is 30.

Part One (Questions 1–12)

(1 mark for each correct answer)
1 Customer Care   7 Oxford MBA
2 CD-ROM   8 caroline@lomas.net.hk
3 $279   9 Park
4 US/United States   10 ten places
5 Programme Office   11 £125
6 Grossman   12 Marketing Manager

Part Two (Questions 13–22)

13 C   18 C
14 B   19 G
15 F   20 D
16 G   21 H
17 D   22 A

Part Three (Questions 23–30)

23 B   27 C
24 C   28 B
25 A   29 C
26 B   30 A

Tapescript

Listening Test Four

Practice Tests for the Cambridge Business English Certificate Level 2. Listening Test 4.

PART 1

Part One. Questions 1 to 12.

You will hear three recorded telephone messages. Write one or two words or a number in the numbered spaces on the forms below.
At the end of each message, rewind the tape and listen again.

Message 1

Message One. Questions 1 to 4.

Look at the form below. You will hear a man ordering some items.

You have 15 seconds to read through the form.

[pause]

Now listen and fill in the spaces.

Man: Yes, um ... I want to order some books and things. The first thing is a book called 'Building Teams'. Oh no, sorry, that's the CD-ROM. It's actually called 'Customer Care' and it's $24.95. Then the CD-ROM. Well, I want two of those and I see that's $100 each but never mind. That's 'Team Building'. No, the other way round, 'Building Teams'. And finally the video about Competitive Strategies which is $279. Thank goodness I only want one of those! Oh, I'm John Hunt and my address is 601 Harmsworth Way, Boston, MA 02163, USA.

I see I'll have to pay a handling charge but as I live in the country that's only $72. Great, thanks.

[pause]

Now rewind the tape and listen again.

[pause]

Message 2

Message Two. Questions 5 to 8.

Look at the form below. You will hear a woman asking for some information.

You have 15 seconds to read through the form.

[pause]

Now listen and fill in the spaces.

Woman: I'm leaving a message for the Oxford Management Programme Office. I think the person I want is David Grossman – G-R-O-S-S-M-A-N? It's Caroline Lomas speaking. Could you send me some information about the Management Programme and the Oxford MBA? The easiest thing is for you get me on my e-mail which is caroline@lomas.net.hk and that's all in lower case. If you need it, my telephone number is 852 235 664485. And my address ...

[pause]

Now rewind the tape and listen again.

[pause]

Message 3

Message Three. Questions 9 to 12.

Look at the form below. You will hear a woman making a booking for an awards ceremony.

You have 15 seconds to read through the form.

[pause]

Now listen and fill in the spaces.

Woman: I saw the advert for your award ceremony at the Park Hotel and I want to book a place. I don't want to book one of those tables with ten places. I just want a seat for one, if that's possible. That's only £125, I hope! I believe that there is someone else from my company booking a table for the senior managers here. Please don't confuse us – I can't afford to pay £1,120! Anyway, my name is Kari Mahmood and I'm the Marketing Manager of Apollo. We are on your mailing list so you'll have the rest of my details. Can you let me know if this is OK?

[pause]

Now rewind the tape and listen again.

[pause]

That is the end of Part One. You now have 20 seconds to check your answers.

[pause]

PART 2

Part Two. Questions 13 to 22.

Section 1

Section One. Questions 13 to 17.

You will hear five people talking about their jobs. For each person, decide which type of job A to H they do.
Write one letter A to H next to the number of the person.
Do not use any letter more than once.

At the end of question 17, rewind the tape and listen again.

You have 15 seconds to read the list of jobs A to H.

[pause]

Now listen and decide what job each speaker does.

[pause]

Question 13 *Thirteen*

Man: It's been a bad day for us today. The art market is extremely sensitive and I'm afraid I expected the picture to go for a lot more. Unfortunately it didn't reach its reserve price and so we are left with a very expensive picture which we have failed to sell. I'm afraid

I have to take responsibility for that sort of thing in my job. I have to take that sort of risk.

[pause]

Question 14 *Fourteen*

Woman: Well, if you want my professional opinion my advice is that in order to avoid paying more tax than you need to you should ensure that your overseas representatives act as consultants to your company. It's better for you if they are not technically your employees. This is especially important as they only work for you on a part-time basis. Now it's quite a different matter if you are planning to open regional offices ...

[pause]

Question 15 *Fifteen*

Man: Finally, thank you for coming here today at such short notice. I hope that by the end of today all staff will be aware of the implications of the take-over and I am relying on you, as my senior managers, to ensure that their concerns and queries are fully answered. It won't be possible to guarantee that their jobs are safe forever, but at least you will be able to reassure them that there will be no redundancies in the next 12 months. Now if you have any questions ...

[pause]

Question 16 *Sixteen*

Woman: I've got three deliveries in the London area and all of those are top priority. However, if you're willing to take a chance, there's a good possibility that I could do a pick up from the airport early this afternoon.

[pause]

Question 17 *Seventeen*

Man: This report has to be on the Minister's desk by Monday morning. I've had the researchers on it for a few weeks and it's looking pretty good. I don't think the Government is going to have too much difficulty as the statistics speak for themselves. There is a clear drop in the unemployment figures, even taking into account seasonal factors.

[pause]

Now rewind the tape and listen again.

[pause]

Section 2

Section Two. Questions 18 to 22.

You will hear another five short pieces. For each piece, decide what task A to H the person is being asked to do. Write one letter A to H next to the number of the piece.

At the end of question 22, rewind the tape and listen again.

You have 15 seconds to read the list of tasks A to H.

[pause]

Now listen and decide what each person has been asked to do.

[pause]

Question 18 *Eighteen*

Woman: I've decided to circulate the report you produced on your visit to Pakistan to the senior management team. Before it goes out, can you make sure that those sales forecasts you put in are as accurate as possible? I suggest you speak to Daniel in Marketing. He's pretty reliable.

[pause]

Question 19 *Nineteen*

Woman: I want you to come to the committee meeting this afternoon. It's going to be quite a tricky one for me so I'll be needing you to make an accurate record of everything that goes on. Of course I'll check it with you afterwards. I know how confusing it can be when everyone seems to be speaking at once!

[pause]

Question 20 *Twenty*

Man: Pam Jones from Human Resources has just called. She wants me to let Mr Easton know that he can start next week. You know, the man who came for an interview last Friday. Trouble is I forgot to ask her what his telephone number is. Still, I suppose it would be better if I put it in writing, don't you think?

[pause]

Question 21 *Twenty-one*

Woman: I'm determined that we are going to get all these consultants' names and details sorted. What I want you to do is to have a word with the IT department and get them to understand what it is we want and then to get them to recommend some specific software. After that you'd better go on some sort of training course so that you'll be able to run it efficiently. Then we'll be in a much better position to find the person we need quickly.

[pause]

Question 22 *Twenty-two*

Man: I've just been in a meeting with some of the staff from finance and you wouldn't believe how disorganised it was. There was no agenda and someone had lost the minutes from the last meeting. Could you put something in writing for me to remind departmental managers that it is not acceptable to hold meetings without the appropriate preparation and follow-up.

[pause]

Now rewind the tape and listen again.

[pause]

That is the end of Part Two.

[pause]

PART 3

Part Three. Questions 23 to 30.

You will hear two people discussing Point of Purchasing (POP) projects.
Choose the best phrase to answer or complete questions 23 to 30.
Mark one letter A, B or C for the phrase you choose.

At the end of the interview, rewind the tape and listen again.

You have 45 seconds to read through the questions.

[pause]

Now listen and mark A, B or C.

[pause]

Man: So what exactly is POP?
Woman: Well, POP stands for Point of Purchasing and it refers to the advertising techniques used to sell specific products at the point where customers buy them.
Man: Such as at the supermarket check-out or on the shelves in a shop?
Woman: Yes, that's right, and managers are slowly beginning to realise how successful it can be and are building it into their general plans for promoting product ranges. The surprising thing is it's taking a while to catch on in a big way.
Man: Is that because firms are going to have to spend a lot of money in the early stages?
Woman: That's true, and of course the displays have to be serviced regularly. But we know that most people don't decide what to buy until they are in the shop. And it seems that retail managers are beginning to see sense at last. Firstly, it's generally accepted that consumers ignore adverts on TV. Secondly, the expansion of cable and satellite TV channels has made it much more difficult to reach all consumers with an effective TV advertising campaign while remaining within budget. Point of Purchasing advertising is more selective but cheaper.
Man: I believe that Samsung, for example, have invested heavily in POP to boost sales of its computer monitors?
Woman: That's right. They wanted to convince consumers to purchase individual components when buying a computer system rather than what it describes as 'inappropriate' packages. They say they have gone for POP because it wasn't just awareness-raising they were after. They wanted to influence even those customers who had decided on something else by demonstrating Samsung's products in store.
Man: So are companies actually employing POP agencies?
Woman: Some are but many, like Ford, are asking their planners to look into the research that has been done in the area to find out things like how long it takes to launch a new brand, how many people visit an advertising fixture in a shop and so on.
Man: But companies are still reluctant to allocate large budgets to POP because it's almost impossible to assess the results of specific campaigns?
Woman: Yes, but there are success stories. The Cheltenham and Gloucester Building Society decided to move into a retail environment and sell their pensions more aggressively. They looked seriously at where they sited displays and did some research to find out where the

Key

best places in the branch were. They placed their leaflets in well-designed dispensers in the walkways between the doors and the counters rather than on the walls.

Man: So you think more companies can be persuaded down the POP route?

Woman: I think retailers will always want to set a number of conditions on POP campaigns. They'll want the campaign to fit in with their store's style and they won't want the products detracting too much from their own brands. They'll also want to manage the area themselves or ensure that the agency keeps the displays in good condition.

Man: So is the future for POP agencies looking good?

Woman: In the short term it's reasonable. The pressure on retail space brought about by retailers' own-label products is an obstacle and

POP needs to develop a more exciting image by using interactive ideas such as smell, visual effects and sound. Hopefully this will mean that consumers stay longer to consider their purchase.

[pause]

Now rewind the tape and listen again.

[pause]

That is the end of Part Three. You now have ten minutes to transfer your answers to your Answer Sheet. [**Teachers:** Time 9 minutes starting now.]

[pause]

You have one more minute.

[pause]

That is the end of the test.

Sample Speaking Test Tapescript

Practice Tests for the Cambridge Business English Certificate Level 2.

This is an example of the Speaking Test.

Interviewer: Good morning. I'm Sheila and this is Frank. He'll just be listening to us.

Inez & Pablo: Good morning.

Interviewer: I'd like to check the spelling of your names. Inez?

Inez: It's I-N-E-Z.

Interviewer: And Pablo?

Pablo: P-A-B-L-O.

Interviewer: Now I'm going to ask you a few questions about yourselves and then we have an activity. Inez, where do you come from?

Inez: I'm from Spain. I live in Madrid at the moment.

Interviewer: What's it like living in Madrid?

Inez: I like it very much. Madrid is an exciting city and there is always lots to do. I go out a lot.

Interviewer: Do you have a job there?

Inez: Yes, I work for a large finance company. I'm a trainee manager for one of the overseas departments.

Interviewer: That sounds interesting. And Pablo, where do you live?

Pablo: Well, for the next few months I'm living in Madrid but I'm hoping to go to Britain to work in the autumn.

Interviewer: And how do you find living in Madrid?

Pablo: It's a good place to be but quite expensive. I'm a student and so I need to be careful with how much I spend. I'm studying business management. I want to go to Britain to work in a bank.

Interviewer: I see, and will you need to speak English in your job?

Pablo: Yes, it'll be very important for me, even though the bank is a Spanish one. So I am studying hard.

Interviewer: Is it the same for you, Inez? Will you need to speak English?

Inez: Yes. It's the same for me. Although the company I work for is Spanish, it does a lot of overseas business, especially in Southeast Asia. Most business with foreigners in that part of the world is done in English. It's a necessity for me to speak and write in English.

Interviewer: Inez, what sort of clothes do you wear?

Inez: When I'm working I have to be very smart so I always wear a skirt and a jacket. The company I work for is in the centre of the city and everyone wears good clothes for the office.

Interviewer: And what about in your free time?

Inez: I like to wear jeans and shirts. I like to be comfortable but I still want to be tidy. I think in Spain people dress well most of the time.

Interviewer: What do you think, Pablo?

Pablo: I agree. The Spanish people are normally well-dressed. Even though I am a student I always wear smart trousers with a belt and a shirt even if I don't wear a tie. In our country I think people notice what you are wearing all the time. They think it matters. I like to look quite smart even if I am just going to classes.

Interviewer: Thank you. Now we are going to move on to the second part of the test. In this activity you are going to find out from each other about two types of overhead projectors. Inez, at the top of your sheet there are some things to find out from Pablo about the Novo Overhead Projector. Ask Pablo for the information. When Inez has finished, Pablo, you will ask her some questions about the

Casco Executive Overhead projector. The information about the projectors is at the bottom of the page. Read through the information carefully. Do you both understand what you have to do?

Inez and Pablo: Yes.

Interviewer: Right, Inez, you begin.

Inez: Pablo, can you tell me how much the projector costs?

Pablo: It costs £497.50.

Inez: And what does it weigh?

Pablo: Oh, it's very light. Only 5.6 kg.

Inez: That's good. Does it have any other extra features?

Pablo: Yes, it has twin lamps and it has a storage, carrying case. Also it folds flat for travelling.

Inez: That sounds very good.

Pablo: Inez, what about the Casco Projector? How big is it?

Inez: Sorry, it does not say exactly how big it is, but it weighs 10.8 kg.

Pablo: Are there any instructions to tell you how to use it?

Inez: Yes, it comes with a user manual.

Pablo: Good. And does it have any extra features?

Inez: Yes. It has a twin fan cooling system and you also get a LCD projection panel, a universal power supply and a remote control.

Pablo: It has a lot of extra things, then.

Inez: Yes.

Interviewer: Now look at the discussion. You have to discuss together which projector is most suitable for you. Remember to include price and weight and anything else you think

is important. You have about 30 seconds to think about it first, then begin.

Pablo: I think the Novo is the best one for me.

Inez: Why is that?

Pablo: Because it is so light and portable. I would like to take it with me when I am travelling. I have to do a lot of travelling so it would be very convenient.

Inez: Yes, I can see it would be the best one for you but I prefer the Casco. It has a lot of useful things like the LCD projection panel. That's very good if I have to give a presentation to a group of people. One of the things I have to do in my job is visit our customers in their organisations and sometimes they don't have very good facilities.

Pablo: But it will be difficult to carry it.

Inez: I know, but I always take an assistant with me and I don't usually have to travel far.

Pablo: But it is expensive. £600 is a lot of money for a projector.

Inez: That depends on how much I use it.

Pablo: That's true. Still, the most important thing for me is that I can easily carry it around with me. I'd like to be able to go to other countries knowing that I have everything I need if I have to give a presentation.

Inez: And for me the most important thing is that I have a good quality projector which will last a long time. So you are going to have the Novo?

Pablo: Yes. And you are going for the Casco?

Inez: Yes.

Interviewer: Thank you Inez and Pablo. That's the end of the test.

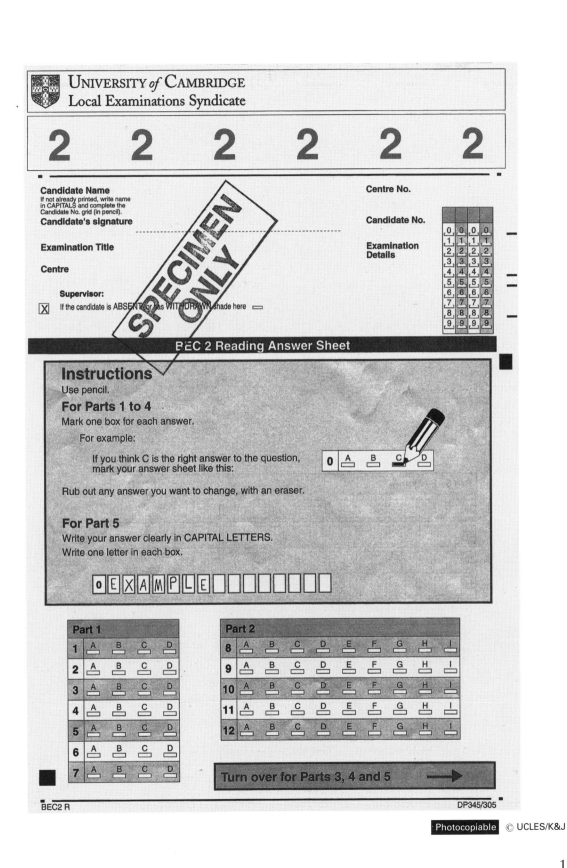

103

Part 3

13	A	B	C	D	E	F	G
14	A	B	C	D	E	F	G
15	A	B	C	D	E	F	G
16	A	B	C	D	E	F	G
17	A	B	C	D	E	F	G
18	A	B	C	D	E	F	G
19	A	B	C	D	E	F	G
20	A	B	C	D	E	F	G

Part 4

21	A	B	C	D
22	A	B	C	D
23	A	B	C	D
24	A	B	C	D
25	A	B	C	D
26	A	B	C	D
27	A	B	C	D
28	A	B	C	D
29	A	B	C	D
30	A	B	C	D
31	A	B	C	D
32	A	B	C	D
33	A	B	C	D
34	A	B	C	D
35	A	B	C	D

Part 5 - Section A

Do not write here

36		1 36 0
37		1 37 0
38		1 38 0
39		1 39 0
40		1 40 0

Part 5 - Section B

Do not write here

41		1 41 0
42		1 42 0
43		1 43 0
44		1 44 0
45		1 45 0

104

2   **2**   **2**   **2**   **2**   **2**

Candidate Name
If not already printed, write name
in CAPITALS and complete the
Candidate No. grid (in pencil).

Candidate's signature

Examination Title

Centre

Supervisor:

☒   If the candidate is ABSENT or has WITHDRAWN shade here ▭

Centre No.

Candidate No.

**Examination
Details**

0	0	0	0
1	1	1	1
2	2	2	2
3	3	3	3
4	4	4	4
5	5	5	5
6	6	6	6
7	7	7	7
8	8	8	8
9	9	9	9

BEC 2 Writing Answer Sheet

Write your answer to Part 1 below

Part 1 (Qu.46)	

Write your answer to Part 2 on the other side of this sheet ➜

This section for use by Examiner only

Q 46	0	1.1	1.2	2.1	2.2	3.1	3.2	4.1	4.2	5.1	5.2

105

Part 2 (Qu.47)

106

UNIVERSITY *of* CAMBRIDGE
Local Examinations Syndicate

2 2 2 2 2 2

Candidate Name
If not already printed, write name
in CAPITALS and complete the
Candidate No. grid (in pencil).

Candidate's signature

Examination Title

Centre

Supervisor:
[X] If the candidate is ABSENT or has WITHDRAWN shade here ▭

Centre No.

Candidate No.

**Examination
Details**

SPECIMEN ONLY

0	0	0	0
1	1	1	1
2	2	2	2
3	3	3	3
4	4	4	4
5	5	5	5
6	6	6	6
7	7	7	7
8	8	8	8
9	9	9	9

BEC 2 Listening Answer Sheet

Instructions
Use pencil
For Part 1
Write your answer clearly in CAPITAL LETTERS.
Write one letter or number in each box.
If the answer has more than one word, leave one box empty between words.
Example:

| 0 | 3 | 0 | | Q | U | E | S | T | I | O | N | S | | | |

For Parts 2 and 3
Mark one box for each answer. Rub out any answer you want to change, with an eraser.

Part 1 - Conversation One

1 | | | | | | | | | | | | | | | | | | | | | | | | | | | | | | | |

1 1 0

2 | | | | | | | | | | | | | | | | | | | | | | | | | | | | | | | |

1 2 0

3 | | | | | | | | | | | | | | | | | | | | | | | | | | | | | | | |

1 3 0

4 | | | | | | | | | | | | | | | | | | | | | | | | | | | | | | | |

1 4 0

Continue on the other side of this sheet ⟶

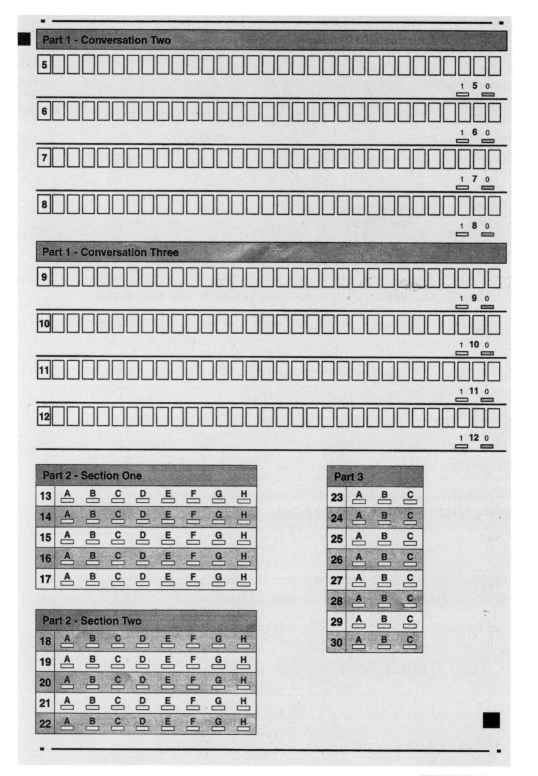

Part 1 - Conversation Two

5

1 **5** 0

6

1 **6** 0

7

1 **7** 0

8

1 **8** 0

Part 1 - Conversation Three

9

1 **9** 0

10

1 **10** 0

11

1 **11** 0

12

1 **12** 0

Part 2 - Section One

13 A B C D E F G H
14 A B C D E F G H
15 A B C D E F G H
16 A B C D E F G H
17 A B C D E F G H

Part 2 - Section Two

18 A B C D E F G H
19 A B C D E F G H
20 A B C D E F G H
21 A B C D E F G H
22 A B C D E F G H

Part 3

23 A B C
24 A B C
25 A B C
26 A B C
27 A B C
28 A B C
29 A B C
30 A B C